ONLY WHEN
IT HURTS

ONLY WHEN IT HURTS

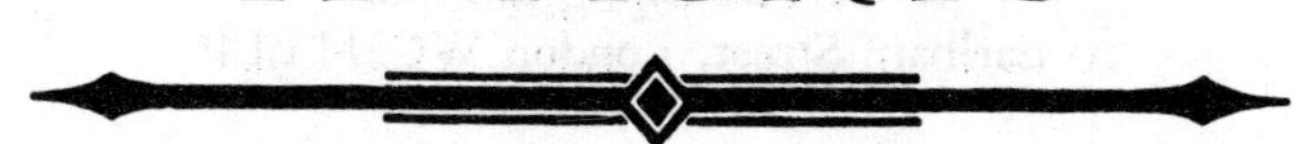

*Being a Curious Collection of
Old Fashioned Remedies and Dissertations
on Matters of Health and Hygiene*

Compiled by
PHYLLIS MORTIMER

WOLFE PUBLISHING

Wolfe Publishing Limited
10 Earlham Street, London WC2H 9LP

SBN 7234 0462 3

Printed in Great Britain by
Oxley Printing Group Ltd, London and Edinburgh

CONTENTS

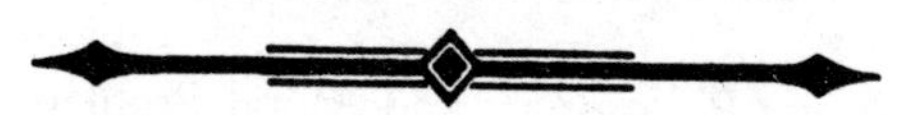

INTRODUCTION

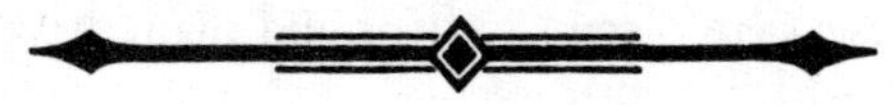

Medicine has changed, and, with increasing momentum, is changing. So is the attitude of doctor to patient and the patient's relationship with his physician. Until recently it has been the custom of Medical Practitioners to hide the secrets of their art from the layman: an undoubted advantage in avoiding any suggestion that knowledge is inadequate or treatment empiric. Nowadays patients wish to know how and why they are treated, and medical information is constantly presented throughout the mass media. It is the natural sequel to the reputable (though often inaccurate) 'Home Medicine' books of the 19th century, which appeared at the same time as numerous and dangerous 'quack' remedy publications.

The purpose of this book is to reveal some of the secrets of the past both to the lay public and doctors alike; with the hope that the extracts selected will amuse, amaze, and sometimes even appal. It may appear that much of the treatment mentioned is painful, inefficient and took up an unnecessary length of time. Indeed it is obvious that a visit to the doctor during the 18th and 19th centuries was hazardous in the extreme. With hindsight criticism is easy, and it is sometimes difficult to understand how patients were able to withstand so much pain and discomfort with apparent philosophic stoicism. However, the impression from contemporary medical literature is that each patient was treated as an individual and the skilled physician was often incredibly accurate in his diagnosis of those conditions which could be determined by the physical examination of his patients.

Only the rich could afford the attentions of a qualified physician or surgeon. For the poor there were three alternatives: to let nature take its course (probably the safest regimen); to join the mass of sick and pitiful humanity at the free clinics, where treatment was usually carried out by inadequately trained students; or to seek help from the numerous charlatans whose wares were readily available. However, in a different class were the herbal remedies which were handed down from generation to generation; these were often excellent and many have formed the basis for modern therapeutic agents.

It is tempting to feel that some of the treatments included here would prove an entertaining improvement on some contemporary clinical therapy. It would be exceedingly unwise to experiment: many of the patients failed to survive the treatment, even when it was orthodox practice!

> Cured yesterday of my disease,
> I died last night of my Physician
> [*Matthew Prior 1664–1721*]

Phyllis M. Mortimer

In Which are Discussed some Fevers and Infectious Diseases

When a man is sick with a fever don't keep on talking to him under the impression that you are doing him good, for you are in all probability worrying him to death. When a man is really ill he doesn't want to be bothered with questions. It is no good asking him where he thinks he got it, or worrying him every moment about how his head feels now. It is easy enough to talk when you are well, but when you've got the ague you've something else to do. Sit down by the bed-side quietly, and if you can help the patient do so, but don't be officious. You must remember that in ague there is often a good deal of irritation of the bladder, and that in certain cases your occasional absence from the room would be desirable.—*The Family Physician*, 1883.

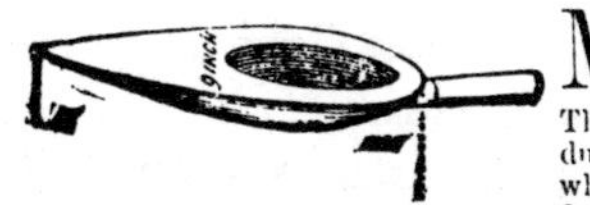

It is very common for some part of the furniture to take frightful shapes in the eyes of a fever patient. Perhaps he may be able to tell you what it is, but if not, by carefully watching the eyes, you will find him looking steadily at one object, and then turn away suddenly, as if he were trying to escape. When these visions are troubling the patient, the best plan, if you can do so, is to remove him into another room. The effect is wonderful. The visions disappear, the dreadful forms are all gone, and the bright and cheerful face tells you better than words what a relief he feels. If you cannot change the room, change the furniture, and if that cannot be done, alter its position.

A singular and yet not uncommon thing in fever with delirium is a strong dislike taken by the patient to a particular person, and this generally not a stranger, but a near relative, one who is greatly beloved by him when in health, and who has been for days and nights watching over him. In some cases this feeling of dislike grows into a hatred so deep that it is not safe to allow the person to remain alone in the room. This is very distressing; it appears so ungrateful, such a poor return for all the care and kindness bestowed upon him, so unnatural, that it is hard to bear.

But it should be remembered that it is unnatural; it is the result of disease, and has no more to do with a patient's real affection than taking a dislike to some particular article of food. As the mind becomes healthy this will pass off; but it is very desirable that the person to whom the dislike is taken should be removed as soon as possible, and not again enter the room till the mind is in a healthier state, or the feeling may become so fixed that it will require a long time to subdue it.—*Till the Doctor Comes*, 1870.

The best plan to adopt with a common Cold, is to restore the proper action of the skin as soon as possible.

Various methods may be used: for instance, a person feels that peculiar warning, which makes him say, 'Now I'm in for a cold, I feel it coming on—headache, chilly, creeping feeling of the skin, and a state of miserableness generally.' If he can manage it, let him go at once and take a Turkish or common vapour bath. Or if he can spare the time, let him go to bed, take ten grains of Dover's powder, with a little sugar, put a large hot bran or oatmeal poultice all over his chest down to the waist, and in an hour after the powder a pint of hot tea, or thin gruel, and an extra blanket or two.

The next morning he should be well rubbed all over with a coarse towel, and take a Seidlitz powder or a large teaspoonful of Epsom salts, either of them, in warm water. But suppose it comes on when business must be attended to. Let him put on an extra quantity of clothing, drink a pint of hot tea, and take a quick walk till the skin is quite damp with perspiration, then cool down gradually. If a person has a cold, not very bad, but what is called 'hanging about them,' a pint of cold water at bedtime, and a little extra bedclothes, will be an excellent remedy without any medicine. But whichever plan you adopt, do not half do it; if you are obliged to give way, do it thoroughly, stay in bed from twelve to twenty-four hours, and give the cold a check. If you are compelled to go out, put on plenty of clothing, work hard at your business, and bustle about as much as possible. —*Till the Doctor Comes*, 1870.

A boil is of no practical value. It is said that everything has its use, but this certainly does not apply to boils. They are of no use; and few people consider them ornamental. They do not improve your personal appearance, and they do not add to your comfort. We are told, on good authority, that in many cases they must be looked upon as salutary, as being the means adopted by Nature to rid the system of morbid matters that irritate the constitution. This may be, but a boil is a violent remedy. Most people, if they had the choice, would prefer a less energetic means of having the system cleared out. Scientific doctors usually call them *furunculi*, but even then they are rather painful.—*The Family Physician*, 1883.

A furred tongue is very common in the case of people who smoke much. This condition always accompanies fever, and is a decided characteristic of that affection. At the same time it must be remembered that for the detection of fever we put our trust in the thermometer, the state of the tongue being of minor importance. When the fur is white, thickish, and tolerably uniform and moist, it usually indicates an open, active state of the fever, in which, though the obvious symptoms may possibly be violent, there is little probability of any lurking mischief, or of a malignant tendency. A yellowish hue of the fur is commonly indicative of disordered liver. A brown or black tongue is a bad sign, usually indicating a low state of the system, and a general condition of depression. Malingerers sometimes manage to simulate the condition by chewing liquorice, tobacco, burnt coffee-grains, and so on.—*Ibid*.

When the pustules of acne *simplex* are few in number, they scarcely deserve any attention, except as symptoms of some constitutional derangement; but when they are considerable, they require the use of different medical measures, as well general as local, on their own account. When the disease appears to be connected with an unsatisfactory discharge of the uterine functions, the treatment must be directed to this object. In young persons of a strong and plethoric constitution, and particularly if about the first appearance of the catamenia, a small bloodletting will afford the most immediate relief; or, if there is pain of the back or loins, a few leeches may be applied to each groin, the feet may be immersed in a warm salt-water pediluvium, and the bowels preserved in an open state by some cooling saline aperient.

The same general treatment is applicable to young male subjects; a small venesection, cooling saline aperients, the powder of sulphur, magnesia, and rhubarb, and, if necessary, a few grains of Plummer's pill, and a course of decoction of taraxacum, with a little sulphate of potass. In both cases, after the aperient and alternative remedies, the diluted *mineral acids* are useful remedies.

The best local application to the eruption in the early stages is decoction of bran, decoction of the seeds of cucumbers or melons, or the emulsion of bitter almonds. It is not until the eruption has declined and become chronic, that gently stimulating applications are required, and they are then of much use. The effect of any irritating lotion used in the early state of the eruption, is to multiply the pustules; but after suppuration, when proportioned to the sensibility of the local affection, they are often of the greatest use. Nor in this period of the disease need there be any apprehension of producing internal disorder by the sudden repulsion of these cutaneous eruptions: it is only in the early and active state of the disease, that headache and disorders of the digestive organs have sometimes been thus produced.—*The Cyclopaedia of Practical Medicine*, 1833.

ERUPTIVE FEVERS

On the fourth or eleventh Day of Eruptive Fever, Spots appear in some, chiefly on the Back, Breast, and Arms, with or without Relief. Some have more, some less, of various Colours, as purple, a brownish livid, or a pale Rose. There are sometimes broad, sometimes small; and in many like Flea-bites. These different Spots serve to distinguish the Fever by several Names, such as miliary, puncticular, bastard petechial, and the like.

When this Disease is at its State, or Vigor, all the Symptoms are worse; the Inquietude runs very high, as well as the Tossing of the Body with unusual Postures. The Mind is disturbed, the Speech incoherent, Sleep wanting, the Sweat is coldish, with a more intense Difficulty of Breathing, and a contracted, unequal, quick and frequent Pulse, as in the nervous Fever.

When a subsultus Tendinum, Want of Thirst, Rumbling in the Belly, Hiccup, an Inflammation of the Fauces from Aphthae, Convulsions, a Syncope, with Coldness of the Extremities, and a most plentiful Sweat supervene to these Symptoms, they are certain Forerunners of Death. On the other hand, when a Sweat breaks out about or on the critical Days, that is the seventh, eleventh, or fourteenth Day, and continues several Days, though Want of Strength remains; or if there is a Looseness for some Days, it is a Sign of Health: And this the more certain, if the contracted Pulse enlarges, the hard grows soft and becomes more equal; if the Patient is more cheerful, and his lying in Bed more sedate, with a Hardness of Hearing, and a turbid Urine, depositing a Sediment. If this happens after the critical Days it is a certain Sign of a happy Event. After this the Sleep, Appetite, and Strength gradually return; but this is seldom the Case before the fourteenth Day.

Patients of a strong Constitution, the common People, and Rustics, with a good Regimen alone, generally succeed better than the weak, timorous, the sad, the thoughtful, the luxurious, the slothful and the studious. All excretions by Urine, Stool or Sweat, are bad in the Beginning, and on other Days except the critical. Those that die are carried off by a Phrensy, or an Inflammation of the Meninges, or of the Oesophagus and Fauces from Aphthae, of the Stomach itself. If Blood is taken away in these Diseases, it is either of a bright red, very fluid and serous, or too thick and blackish.

In the Cure of this Disease, the Physician should take Care not to disturb the salutary Excretions, but proceed cautiously, and abstain from strong Medicines of every Kind, watching and assisting the Motions of Nature as much as possible.

To raise the Spirits and restore the Strength, a little Wine will not be improper, with Harts-horn Jellies, China Orange, or Seville Orange Juice with Sugar.

A congruous Regimen in these Diseases is of very great Consequence; for if the Patient is kept too hot, the Dissolution of the Blood will be promoted, a Costiveness will be induced, the Anxiety will be increased, the impure salt, acrid Humours will be actuated, the Strength will be exhausted, the Sweating will be too speedy and profuse, and Spots will appear on the Skin. On the other hand, if Cold is incautiously admitted, especially to the Feet, Perspiration will be checked, the Eruptions and Spots will be driven back: There will be griping Pains, a Looseness, and the critical Evacuations will be disturbed. All sudden Changes from hot to cold, or cold to hot, are equally bad. A temperate Regimen is left.

The Perspiration should constantly be kept up, and the Linen of any kind should not rashly be changed, nor should the Patient be removed from one Bed to another. He should be enjoined not to rise frequently, nor should the Bed be made on critical Days, when the Spots are likely to appear. And if the Bed-clothes are wet and must needs be changed, let them be well aired and pretty much worn. A Night or Bed-gown will be also very proper to keep on constantly; for it will be a Defence against cold Air.

The Mind should be kept as cheerful as possible, and all Occasions shunned of exciting Anger, Fear, Terror, or Pusill-animity in the Patient. His Hope of Recovery should be kept up as much as possible, instead of being terrified with the Prediction of Death. I have known Patients who have laboured under this Disease, and would in all Probability have recovered, if some Priest or over-wise Physician had not foretold and inculcated a speedy Death; which has so affected the sick Person with Dread and Horror, that there has been an immediate Change manifestly for the worse.—*The General Practice of Physic,* 1763.

OF THE SLOW AND HECTIC FEVER

Fevers from Disorders in the Hypochondria. When the Patient is plethoric, and cacochymical, cachectical, scorbutical, or the Menses, or Haemorrhoidal Evacuations are stopped, and cause this Disease; or if it proceed from Voraciousness, or bad Diet, or the Abuse of spirituous Liquors; then Endeavours must be used to free the Liver, Spleen, and Mesentery, and its Vessels and

Glands from Obstructions. For this purpose, Mineral Waters are proper, as the Seltzers, likewise the Thermae, or hot Bath Waters.

But where these cannot be had, I have used with Success, a Decoction of thin Veal Broth, with the Roots of Succory, Fennel, Asparagus, Dog-Grass and Viper-Grass; the Patient is to drink a Quart a Day for some weeks, taking before it some Preparation of Steel, such as the Tincture of Steel, or the Tincture of Martial Flowers.

Fevers from an Erosion of the Stomach and Bowels. When a slow Fever happens from an Erosion of the Stomach and Bowels, all sharp, salt, acid, stimulating Things are as bad as Poison. I have known a Decoction of Sassafras and Cortex Eleutheriae, in Milk, as also of Camomile Flowers, and the Tops of Yarrow, drank to about a Quart to a Day, very serviceable; likewise Roots of Marsh-Mallows, or Rice boiled in Milk; or Gum Dragant dissolved in Mint-Water. Milk Clysters are also beneficial, with the Yolk of an Egg. Turpentine and Honey, or other Emollients, with the Syrup of Marsh-Mallows. When there are Spasms in the Bowels, our antispasmodic Pills are useful, made of Extract of Camomile, Yarrow, Oil of Nutmegs, Extract of Saffron, and Castor.

Fever from the Loss of the necessary Fluids, and Want of Strength. When this Fever proceeds from excruciating Passions of the Mind, Sadness, Cares, hard Labour, Watching, Abstinence, inordinate Coition, the Fluor Albus, Gonorrhaea, Diarrhoea, giving suck too long, or running Ulcers, from which the Strength and viscid Juices are decayed, all Things that raise a Commotion in the Blood, and stimulate the Bowels, are bad; as also Aliment that is too substantial. It rather requires Rest both of Body and Mind, a light temperature Diet, Medicines that sheath the Acrimony, allay the Heat, and gently raise the sinking Spirits.

Hence, Emulsions of Almonds, of the four Cold Seeds are proper; as also Ass's, Goat's, or Woman's Milk, with the Juice of River-cresses; Chicken-Broth, Broth made of River-Crabs, or Wood-snails bruised; some commend Oysters, if the Stomach will bear them, and Instances of their extraordinary Efficacy have been produced. But little Wine should be allowed, and that of the softest Kind, mixed with Water.

Fevers from the Abuse of Spirituous Liquors. In this Case all heating Spirituous Liquors, and Strong Beer should be avoided; as also Analeptics, Inciders of Phlegm, and Stomachics. Gruel, after Lower's Method, will be proper, made of Oatmeal, Succory-Root, red Poppy-Flowers, and a little stibiated Nitre; likewise Whey, with a little Nitre, or fresh Buttermilk, which is greatly esteemed for its extraordinary Efficacy; to these we may add, Ptisans of Pearl-Barley and Succory, thin Emulsions and Hart's-horn Jellies.

Fevers from a Suppression of the Menses. This Circumstance requires immediate Bleeding in the Foot and resolvent Decoctions of Succory-Roots, Leaves of Sow-thistle, Daisy and Elder-flowers, forbearing all strong Emmenagogues. But if the Patient has laboured long under a slow or Hectic Fever, and is greatly weakened and emaciated, Bleeding must be omitted.

If after Lying-in the Menses are stopped, and there is a Hectic with an Atrophy, Cough, Diarrhoea, universal Languor of the whole Body, and a slow consuming Heat, no Emmenagogues must be used, but directly the contrary. The same may be said of the Stoppage of the periodical Flux of the Bleeding-Piles, for the giving of Aloetics in this Case has hurried many out of the World.

Fevers from a Marasmus Senilis. There are two Causes which produce tabetic Fevers in Persons advanced in Years; the one is a Plethora, or rather a Quantity of thick Blood stuffing and obstructing the Viscera and the Mesentery: The other, a Cacochymy, from a Plenty of impure salt Serum, not secreted through the Skin, or otherwise.

If the Patient has been addicted to a sedentary inactive Life, his Appetite remaining good, and has omitted accustomary Bleeding, or the spontaneous Evacuations of Blood are ceased, and he is in Danger of a slow Hectic, Bleeding is indicated and wholesome.—*The General Practice of Physic,* 1763.

OF THE CATARRHAL FEVER

Catarrhal Fever more frequently attacks Women and Children than Men, and those that indulge themselves in strong Liquors.

It sometimes happens from the drying up of a scald Head and other Eruptions. Sometimes it is epidemical, and proceeds from a subtile caustic Matter in the Air. When it is attended with a sudden Loss of Strength it is of a malignant Nature.

This Disease is most frequent in the Spring and Autumn, in sudden Changes of the Weather from hot to cold, from dry to moist, and vice versa; as also from Change of Air, if of different Qualities; from being exposed to the cold Air of the Night, and from throwing off Winter-Garments too soon. Sometimes it is epidemical and contagious.

This Disease is not dangerous in itself, if rightly managed, and terminates in seven or fourteen Days at farthest, for the Lassitude of the Body then disappears: And the other Complaints, especially the Head-ach and Hemicrania are appeased, when the Catarrh appears, and there is a plentiful Discharge from the Nostrils.

The Intentions of Cure are three. 1. To sheath the Acrimony of the Lympha. 2. To increase Perspiration. 3. To promote the Expectoration of the viscid Mucus.

The saline Sharpness of the Lympha may be taken off by the absorbent and diaphoretic Powders, humecting and oleous Remedies, such as Oil of Sweet Almonds, Sperma Ceri, Milk, Cream, Almond-Emulsions, with the Addition of white Poppy Seeds, Barley-Broth, Water-Gruel, Chicken-Broth, with the Yolk of an Egg. As also Liquorice-Juice, Liquorice-Tea, dried Figs and Raisins. If the Acrimony is very subtile and corroding, gentle Anodynes should take place, such as Saffron, Diacodium, and Storax Pills.

To promote Perspiration, order Tea, with Leaves of Veronica (Male Speedwell), Hyssop, Liquorice-Root, Elder-Flowers, wild Poppies, and Fennel-Seeds. As also the more fixed Diaphoretic Powders, with antispasmodic Waters; but especially bodily Motion and Exercise.

To promote the Excretion of the thick, viscid Mucus, Figs and Raisins are proper, with Brandy burnt, and reduced almost into a Syrup. Likewise a pectoral Elixir, made of Gum Ammoniac, Myrrh, Liquorice-Root, Elecampane-Root, Saffron, Beaujamin, and Oil of Aniseed, whose Virtue may be heightened by the vinous Spirit of Sal Ammoniac or Tincture of Tartar. The stagnating Mucus of the Nose, may be dissolved by often holding to the Nose the dry volatile Sal Ammoniac, mixt with a few Drops of genuine Oil of Marjaram.

The Regimen should be temperate, and cooling Things as well as Acids should be avoided; Opiates are not convenient, when the Head is weak and heavy, the Body costive, and the Age far advanced.

The Ailment should be sparing, the Drink warm and wholesome; the best is a Decoction of Pearl-Barley and Shavings of Harts-horn; as also Water-Gruel. Wine is not proper till the Decline of the Disease.

If the Heat is intense and the Constitution bilious, a few Grains of Nitre may be added to the diaphoretic Powders, and the Emulsions may be taken more freely.

If the Body is costive, besides, Water Gruel, Manna, Prunes, and Raisins, nothing is better than an emollient Clyster. Or the Patient may take at Night, going to Bed, half a Dram of the Aromat Pills, with four Grains of Storax Pills, which will open the Body, and appease the Cough.

In the Decline of the Disease, when the Cough is too moist, the Defluxion great and obstinate, it will be proper to take a large Dose of Manna to two or three Ounces in Fennel-water, to carry the Humours downward. To which Purpose also, a Scruple or half a Dram of Rufus's Pills may be given. Cathartics are hurtful in the Beginning.

When the Cough is very violent, it must be appeased with a Mixture of Oil of Sweet Almonds, fresh drawn, and French Syrup of Capillaire, or the following *Electary.—Ibid.*

OF EPIDEMIC, CATARRHAL FEVERS

When there is a Pain in the Head with a Delirium, cut open a live Chicken or Pigeon, and apply it to the Head when the Hair is shaved off. In Fainting, Vomiting, the Cardialgia or extreme Lowness, apply a Plaister of Venice Treacle, expressed Oil of Nutmegs, Camphire, Balsam of Peru, Saffron, Oil of Juniper, and a little Spirit of Wine to the Region of the Praecordia; as also in a Hiccup, (but more especially a musk Bolus.) In Dryness and Heat of the Fauces, direct Harts-horn Jellies with Juice of Lemons and Sugar-Candy, or Syrup of Mulberries. Likewise, let the Mouth be washed with a Decoction of Figs, Syrup of Mulberries and Nitre. When the Patient is very sleepy, let the Legs and Soles of the Feet be washed with Vinegar of Rue, or apply a mild Blister to the Calves of the Legs.—*Ibid.*

2

Of Inflictions of the Mind and Disturbances of the Emotions

OF MELANCHOLY AND MADNESS

Melancholy and Madness may be very properly considered as Diseases nearly allied; for we find they have both the same Origin; that is, an excessive Congestion of Blood in the Brain: They only differ in Degree, and with Regard to the Time of Invasion. Melancholy may be looked upon as the primary Disease, of which Madness is only the Augmentation.

When Persons begin to be melancholy, they are sad, dejected, and dull, without any apparent Cause; they tremble for Fear, are destitute of Courage, subject to Watching, and fond of Solitude; they are fretful, fickle, captious and inquisitive; sometimes niggardly to an Excess, and sometimes foolishly profuse and prodigal. They are generally costive, and when they discharge their Excrements they are often dry, round, and covered with a black, bilious Humour. Their Urine is little, acrid and bilious; they are troubled with Flatulences, putrid and fetid Eruptations. Sometimes they vomit an acrid Humour with Bile. Their Countenances become pale and wan; they are lazy and weak, and yet devour their Victuals with Greediness.

Those who are actually mad, are in an excessive Rage when provoked to Anger. Some wander about; some make a hideous Noise; others shun the sight of Mankind; others, if permitted, would tear themselves to pieces. Some, in the highest Degree of the Disorder, see red Images before their Eyes, and fancy themselves struck with Lightning. They are so salacious, that they have no Sense of Shame in their venereal Attempts. When the Disease declines, they become stupid, sedate, and mournful, and sensibly affected with their unhappy Situation.

The antecedent Signs are a Redness and Suffusion of the Eyes with Blood; a tremulous and inconstant Vibration of the Eyelids; a Change of Disposition and Behaviour; Supercilious Looks, a haughty Carriage, disdainful Expressions, a Grinding of the Teeth, unaccountable Malice to particular Persons. Also little Sleep, a violent Head-ache, Quickness of Hearing, a Singing of the Ears; to these may be added incredible strength, Insensibility of Cold, and, in Women, an accumulation of Blood in the Breasts, in the Increase of this disorder.

It may also arise from violent Love in either Sex, especially if attended with Despair; from profuse Evacuations of the Semen; from an hereditary Disposition; from narcotic and stupefactive Medicines; from previous Diseases, especially acute Fevers. Violent Anger will change Melancholy into Madness; and excessive Cold, especially of the lower Parts, will force the Blood to the Lungs, Heart, and Brain; whence oppressive Anxieties, Sighs and Shortness of Breathing; Tremors and Palpitations of the Heart; thus Vertigoes and a Sensation of Weight in the Head; Fierceness of the Eyes; long Watchings; various Workings of the Fancy, intensely fixed upon a single Object, are produced by these Means. To these may be added a Suppression of usual Haemorrhages, and omitting customary Bleeding: hence Melancholy is a Symptom very frequently attending hysteric and hypochondriac Disorders.—*The General Practice of Physic*, 1763.

Trembling is an involuntary Shaking, chiefly of the Hands and Head, sometimes of the Feet, sometimes of the Tongue and Heart. It is a Disorder which frequently attacks Persons advanced in Years, and sometimes the younger Sort. It seems to arise from a Defect of the Spirits; sometimes from Terror, and sometimes from a Plethora. Too much drinking of Coffee will produce a Trembling in some Persons, as plentiful Drinking and Surfeiting will in others. The Cure is difficult in all.

Trembling will sometimes happen from great Passions of the Mind, especially Anger; but this is accidental. Those that dig in Mines, and work about Metals, are pretty often subject to a Tremor.

Trembling is sometimes dangerous, because it degenerates into other nervous Distempers, as a Spasm, Palsy, Lethargy, Apoplexy; in old People it is incurable.

In the Cure, those Things should be avoided that promote the Diseaes, and the Patient should drink Balm or Sage Tea, or a Diet-drink made with China Root, and the same Ingredients; or Peruvian Bark may be taken, with the Infusion of Balm or Sage, or succinated Spirits of Hartshorn, twice or thrice in a Day, and in the Evening an antispasmodic Powder may be taken, especially if the Patient be hot or uses much Wine.

Outwardly, the Neck and Spine of the Back may be rubbed with the Spirits of Ants, Earth-worms, and Sal Ammoniac, mixed together; a fourth Part of the volatile Spirits will be sufficient, or Opodeldoc may be used in their stead.

If the Patient is plethoric, Bleeding is useful; and, in old Persons, a Draught of generous Wine at Meals. Pediluvia, hot Baths, and other mineral Waters may be carefully used.—*Ibid.*

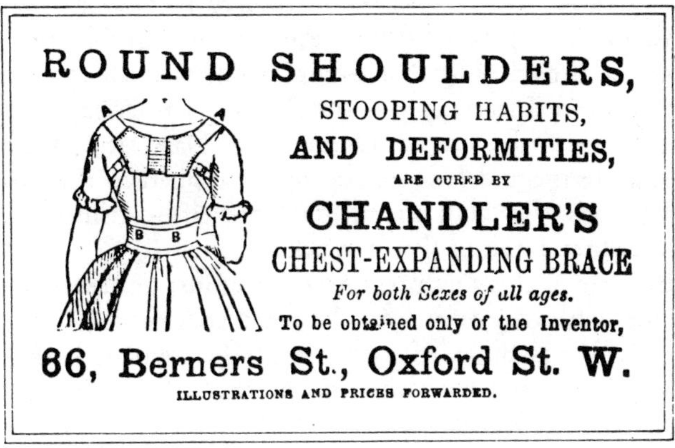

OF A DEFECT OF THE MEMORY

The remote Causes of Defects of the Memory are Hurts of the Head, Falls, Contusions, Passions of the Mind, and certain Things taken inwardly, acute Diseases, especially the Epilepsy and Melancholy.

If the Memory is suddenly hurt, without any external Cause, it is a Forerunner of an Apoplexy. If it proceeds from malignant acute Diseases, or Poisons, it is incurable.

With Regard to the Cure; if the Spirits are too fervid, they are to be appeased; if torpid, they must be excited with Aromatics. The general Remedies are Cubebs eaten fasting (but young People must not be too busy with them) Castor, Amber, and all Spirituous Aromatics. Externally, Oil of Myrrh should be applied to the Temples and Vertex; if the Fluids are abundant and cold, Pepper infused in Wine is good, and Aromatics in general.—*Ibid.*

Almonds, Decoction of Scorzonera-Roots, Almond Cream, and Winter-Flummery, used as Aliment; likewise Tea made of Cowslip Flowers, and gentle Laxatives. When the Patient is restless and wakeful, the Night before a Crisis, no Hypnotics should be given.

Sleepiness may proceed from any Cause which hinders the free Flux and Reflux of the Spirits, from the Marrow of the Brain through the Nerves to the Organs of the Senses, and the Muscles which are governed by the Will, and from hence back to the Origin of these Nerves, and the medullary Part of the Brain; all these Causes may proceed from a Plethora and an Obstruction or Effusion of the Humours, a Compression and Inflammation, a Gangrene, and Inactivity of the Vessels, a Collapsion from Inanition, from the use of Opium and Narcotics, Aromatics, spirituous, fermented Liquors too much applied to the Nostrils, or taken into the Body, hard, fat, plentiful Aliment, which remains a long Time in the Stomach.

In the Cure of this Disorder, Attention must be always given to the Cause; when the Spirits are deficient, they must be increased; if the Motion is disorderly, they must be regulated, that they may flow freely and without Impediment; all Hindrances must be removed; the Organs which are hurt must be restored, and the debilitated parts must be strengthened.

In Fevers, when the Patient is almost continually dozing, sharp Clysters are to be injected, Blisters are to be laid on, and Cataplasms of Herrings or Horse-Radish must be applied to the Soles of the Feet. If the Countenance is red, and the Eyes are inflamed, it is best cured by Bleeding and relaxing the Belly.—*Ibid.*

OF THE EPILEPSY

The Epilepsy is extremely difficult to be cured in Adults, but in Children it is the reverse. Blisters laid to the back Part of the Head are of great Use, a little before the Paroxysm is expected: and the Time may more certainly be foreknown, as this Disease is influenced by the Moon, and attends upon its Phases, especially the New or Full Moon. The most proper Medicines to correct the Juices seem to be Native Cinnabar and wild Valerian Root.

A Dram of which may be given Morning and Evening for three or four Months, and afterwards, two or three Days before the New and Full.—*Ibid.*

OF ST. VITUS'S DANCE

St Vitus Dance is most commonly a slight Evil, and generally seizes weak Habits of Body; Girls more frequently than Boys, and seldom Adults. Wherefore I never found it difficult to be cured by the cold Bath and chalybeate Medicines. Some Physicians have tried in vain to cure these Disorders by Sydenham's Method, for want of attending to their periodical Return, according to the Phases of the Moon. I knew a lusty Girl, about five Years of Age, whose Convulsions were so strong and frequent, that her Life was almost despaired of; after Evacuations, and other Medicines, she continued well for a few Days, but was seized again at the full Moon with a most violent Fit: After this, the Disease kept pace with the Tides; she lay speechless during the whole Time of Flood, and recovered upon the Ebb, This continued till the New Moon; then a dry Scab, the Consequence of a Blister on the Crown of her Head broke, from whence ran a considerable Quantity of limpid Serum, and this Running being encouraged, the Fits returned no more. However, I ordered her three or four Purges with Mercurius Dulcis, about the New and Full of the Moon.—*Ibid.*

OTHER CONVULSIVE DISORDERS

As to the Cure of other Convulsive Disorders, if the Patient is plethoric, or the Pulse great, it must be begun with Bleeding, either in the Arm or Foot; and, if occasion require, it must be repeated two or three Times, but not till the Fit is over. The Air should be dry and serene, with constant Exercise; the Aliment should be easy of Digestion, and all hot spirituous Liquors should be avoided. The constant Drink should be the Decoction of Scorzonera Roots, with Shavings of Hartshorn, or Whey, or the Seltzers Mineral Waters. Pedilavia are likewise proper of River-water, Wheat-Bran, and Chamomile Flowers. They should be used pretty warm and deep, at the Time of going to Bed, and afterwards Sweating should by promoted.

I have known convulsive Disorders cured by the free Use of cold Water alone.

If, about the Time of Puberty, this Disease proceeds from too early or excessive Coition, or violent Passions of the Mind, all Things which cause a Commotion in the Fluids must be avoided, such as, Aromatics, sharp Purges, Emetics, spirituous Liquors, inordinate Motions of the Body or Mind, and all heating Things in general. On the contrary, the Diet should be soft, emollient, and nourishing; such as Cow's or Ass's Milk, or Whey; as also Baths of sweet Water mixed with Milk. Likewise Jellies, and Decoctions of Scorzonera, Barley, Hartshorn, Ivory Shavings, and Viper's Flesh for ordinary Drink, and Chocolate.—*Ibid.*

If a woman is seized with involuntary and alternate weeping and laughter, with heaving and distressed breathing, the face should be shocked with large dashes of cold water, and at the same time the back of the head should be thoroughly wetted and the nape of the neck rubbed with a frequently renewed cold wet towel. Having done this for three or four minutes, let her lie down and let a very strong pressure be made upon the chest in order to suspend the labouring respiration. Whilst doing this let the hands be rubbed in very cold water for five or eight minutes; and simultaneously with this, let the soles of the feet be rubbed with strong mustard and water. If it be possible to reach the belly, apply a cold wet thick-folded towel all over it. The persevering employment of these measures in succession will rarely fail to shorten an hysterical paroxysm. The pressure on the chest, stronger and heavier than the woman could bear in her ordinary state, gives the greatest relief to the breathing: whilst the various shocks given by the other processes disperse the disordered circulation in the spine upon which the morbid phenomena depend; as all the remedies are applied to nerves which take their immediate source in it. Stimulating odours may be applied to the nerves of the nostril with the same view: but I have not generally found them to be necessary.—*A Guide to Domestic Hydrotherapeia*, 1863.

We should suspect a person if he could not speak, and yet could swallow and write well. The impostor nearly always pretends to be absolutely dumb, and seldom knows enough about his pretended complaint to see the necessity of uttering some word or word-like syllable, as the true aphasic nearly always does. This reminds us of the case of a soldier who, with the view of obtaining his discharge, pretended that he had been suddenly struck dumb. He was taken to the doctor, who at once suspected the real nature of the case. The man was told to try and say 'Ah', it being explained to him that he would have no difficulty as it was 'a purely laryngeal sound, unconnected with the faculty of language.' The effort was successful. He was then told to say 'No,' which, it was explained, was 'a sound of similar character.' Not seeing the trap, he promptly replied as directed, 'No.' 'Well, my friend,' said the doctor, 'if you can say "No" you can say anything; so good day.'—*The Family Physician*, 1883.

Ecstasy is not a common complaint, but still many cases have been recorded even during the last five or six years. One of the best known is that of Louise Lateau, who was born at Bois de Haine, a small village in Belgium, in the year 1850. Even as a child she exhibited symptoms of nervous derangement. We are told that she loved solitude and silence, and spent most of her time in meditation and prayer. She was subject to paroxysms of ecstasy, during which she spoke on the subjects of charity, poverty, and the priesthood. She fancied that she was St. Ursula, St. Roch, St. Theresa, and the Holy Virgin. Bleeding, or 'stigmatisation,' as it is called, appeared soon after the onset of these seizures. One Friday she bled from the left side of her chest; on the following Friday the flow was renewed and, in addition, blood escaped from the backs of both feet; whilst on the third Friday not only did she bleed from the side and feet, but also from the backs and palms of both hands. This continued for a long time, and finally other bleeding points were established between the shoulders and on the forehead. The evidence seemed to show that there was *bona fide* bleeding, and that it was not the result of a wound made artificially. In addition to these phenomena, Louise declared that she never slept, that she had had nothing to eat or drink for four years, that she had not had a fæcal evacuation for three years and a half, and that the urine was utterly suppressed. This was undoubtedly untrue.

On being closely interrogated she admitted that, though she did not sleep, she had short periods of forgetfulness at nights—a distinction without a difference. One of the doctors who investigated the case, on suddenly opening a cupboard in her room, found that it contained fruit and bread. It was also shown that her chamber communicated directly with a yard at the back of the house, so that it was perfectly possible for her to have slept, eaten, defæcated and urinated to her heart's content without any one being a bit the wiser. Quite a number of books have been written about this interesting young lady, the theologians endeavouring to prove that she was the subject of miraculous intervention, and the doctors regarding her simply in the light of a curious case of ecstasy. We have very little doubt that bromide of potassium would soon have put a stop to the phenomena. Systematic watching would have been attended with the same result as in the case of the Welsh fasting-girl, or with a sudden restoration of appetite.

Sometimes ecstasy occurs as an epidemic; the strange spasmodic epidemics of the Middle Ages were undoubtedly of this nature. A few years ago an epidemic of ecstasy or emotional exhibitions occurred in several parish churches in one of the most northerly of the Shetland Islands. It was brought to an abrupt conclusion by a rough fellow of a kirk officer, who carried out a troublesome patient and 'tossed her into a wet ditch.' From that time forth no more cases occurred. This is not the only instance in which epidemics of this nature have been arrested by arguments addressed to the fears of the subjects. Making preparations to cauterise the region of the spine with a red-hot iron has often a most beneficial effect.—*Ibid.*

3

Of Conditions of the Urine and Passage of the Stone

Urine on standing often throws down a pinkish deposit. You may often find it at the bottom of your chamber, especially on a cold winter morning. If you empty some of your hot shaving water into it you will find that it will quickly disappear, and the same will happen if you put it before the fire, supposing that you are Sybaritic enough to have one in your bed-room. This deposit consists of what is known as urates or lithates. If you took the trouble to examine it under the microscope—which you will not—you would find that it was quite structureless, not crystalline, or anything of that kind. The deposit in the urine of lithates is no sign of kidney disease, but its frequent occurrence is to be regarded as an indication of liver disorder, arising from causes sometimes temporary, at others more or less permanent. Persons who enjoy the best of health are liable to deposits of lithates in the urine after a surfeit of food, or even after partaking moderately of one of the fashionable dinners of the age.—*The Family Physician*, 1883.

OF THE FLUIDS WHICH PROCEED FROM THE BLOOD

As it is a good Sign when the Urine is thick, and deposites a Sediment in Fevers, so, on the contrary, if there is no Sediment in intermitting Fevers, but the Urine continues clear, and lets fall no Sediment in the cold Fit, it is a bad Sign. If after the Fit it has no Sediment, but is pellucid, it is an exceeding bad Sign. In all inflammatory Fevers, if the Urine is clear and of a purple Colour, or brown and of a deep Colour, frothy and without Sediment, it is an ill Token: Likewise it is always observed, that in a continual Fever, if the Urine is turbid, and does not grow clear, either by the Fire or Rest, nor deposits a Sediment, it is a very dangerous Presage; it is likewise very bad, when in continual Fevers, it is thick on the first Days, and in the Remainder, especially the critical Days, it is thin and without Sediment.

In the Decline of catarrhal Fevers, and in the Small-pox and Measles, if the Urine from clear and aqueous, becomes thick and high-coloured, with a Sediment, it is a certain Sign that the Disease remits.

In Consumptions and all other violent and chronical Diseases, if the Urine is thick, little, high-coloured, and of a dark Red, with a copious Sediment, and a Fatness swimming on it, which adheres to the Sides of the Urinal, the Body at the same time wasting away, it is a Sign of a slow hectic Fever, which is generally fatal. The like Danger is threatened, when, in dropsical Persons, the Urine is like that of Hectics; for its Scarcity is a Sign that the Lympha is extravasated into some Cavity or porous Substance; and, if the Colour is of a deep Red, with a gross Sediment, it shews that the intestine Motion and Heat dissolves the Blood, and that the Liver is obstructed, whence a bilious Sordes is separated therefrom.

Sometimes the Urine is united with an oily Matter, and made without Noise, having various Colours on the Surface, chiefly bluish, and adheres so strongly to the Sides of the Urinal, that it cannot be washed off even with a lixivious Liquor. This is a Sign of a Colliquation of the Fat. Silvius gives an Instance of a young Woman, who had it like Butter; and Fernelius mentions a Man, who, in eight Days, was reduced from a large Size to be very slender, without any other Disease; it shews a Consumption, an Atrophy, and an Hectic. Sometimes this is observable in Fevers, and the oleous Matter is more plentiful, in Proportion to the Fatness of the Body.

When the Urine abounds too much with a tartareous Matter, which is known by its adhering to the Sides of the Chamber-pot, it is a Sign of a Disposition to the Gravel and Stone. When there is small Sand in the Urine, it shews those Disorders to be actually present. Sometimes shining yellow Crystals are seen on the Sides of the Pot, which is a Sign of arthritic or rheumatic Pains. When the Urine is bloody or whitish, from a Mixture of Pus, or loaded with a glutinous, thick, tenacious Matter, of a bad Smell, which sinks to the Bottom, and does not dissolve by the Agitation of the Vessel, it is a certain Sign of an Ulcer in the Kidneys or Bladder; sometimes in the Stone and Ulcer of the Bladder, it is like the White of an Egg, and so tenacious, that it will not divide, but falls from the Vessel like a Mass of Jelly.—*The General Practice of Physic*, 1763.

Diabetes Mellitus. This is the commoner form, and the one which is usually meant when the term diabetes alone is used. If you are suffering from diabetes, and yet have no sugar in your urine, this is not your complaint. You must pass on to diabetes insipidus. Urine containing sugar differs strikingly in many particulars from healthy urine. It is commonly of a light colour, and being so copious is usually free from any deposit. Its odour is somewhat peculiar, and is said by some to resemble sweet hay, and by others to be like the faint smell of an apple-chamber. Moreover, its taste is more or less decidedly sweet. If you just dip your finger into ordinary healthy urine, and put it to the tip of your tongue, you find that it is tasteless, or very nearly so; but if you do this to urine containing sugar, *you*, naturally enough, perceive that it is sweet. Sugar in the urine occasionally testifies its presence in other ways. Sometimes it undergoes a kind of rude crystallisation as the urine dries. A girl who suffered from this complaint observed that if her water were accidentally spilt upon her black stuff shoes every drop left a white powdery spot behind it. In another instance the patient was first alarmed by finding that her black worsted stockings were sticky and covered with a white dust, from the same cause. In still another case the patient's attention was first drawn to his urine by the number of flies and wasps which its sweetness attracted to the chamber-pot. It is said that in India the red ants have been observed to swarm in the same way about a vessel containing diabetic urine.

There is a very simple and beautiful test, by means of which the presence of sugar in the urine may be detected. A few crumbs of German yeast are put into the bottom of a small, narrow-necked bottle; this is filled up to the brim with the suspected urine, covered with a saucer, and then inverted. If a little urine be put in the saucer and the bottle be kept upright, the fluid will not run out. The saucer and inverted bottle should then be placed on one side in a warm place—say on the mantel-piece. If sugar be present fermentation takes place, giving rise to carbonic gas, which forces out of the bottle the whole or a portion of the urine. There is one precaution which should be observed. Some specimens of yeast spontaneously evolve bubbles of gas, so that it is desirable to perform a similar experiment with simple water in the place of the urine, and to compare the results.—*The Family Physician, 1883.*

Urinary calculi vary exceedingly in their size, form, and tenacity. Some calculi do not equal a millet-seed in size, while others have been found so large as to fill up the entire cavity of the bladder. Mr Earle has described a very large stone which had been extracted, but with a fatal result, by the celebrated Cheselden. Its weight was $18\frac{1}{2}$ ounces, its circumference in the large axis was $11\frac{1}{4}$ inches, in its short axis 10 inches. Dr Charles Preston relates in the Philosophical Transactions, that he saw, at La Charité, in Paris, a stone which weighed 51 ounces. The patient died under the hands of the operator. Mr Harmer, of Norwich, extracted from the bladder a stone which weighed 15 ounces and had a diameter of $4\frac{3}{4}$ inches by $3\frac{1}{2}$. The patient recovered, but a fistulous opening remained. In the case of Sir David Ogilvie, Mr Cline performed the operation, but could not extract the stone. After death it was found to measure 16 inches in its longest diameter, and 14 in its shortest, and to weigh 44 ounces. The Breslau collection contains an account of a stone found in the bladder after death, which weighed 72 ounces. Kesselning relates that he saw, in Moraud's Museum at Paris, a stone which weighed 6 pounds 3 ounces; and the model of another which was still larger.—*The Cyclopaedia of Practical Medicine, 1833.*

Mrs Stephen's Medicine for the Stone, as communicated to the Publick by her, is a Composition operose and troublesome, several Parts of it being of little or no Use, and others plainly calculated to disguise the rest. The Ingredients of which it consists have been examined by Dr Hales, and Dr Hartley, who have with much Judgment rejected the superfluous Parts, and reduced this pompous Medicine to a slacken'd Powder of calcin'd Egg-Shells, and a Solution of Soap, in the following Form:
Let two Scruples, two and a half, or a Dram of Egg-shells (calcin'd until they acquire a pungent fiery Taste, and from being black, become white again; and afterwards expose to a dry Air for a Month, six Weeks, or two Months', that is, 'till they slacken

or fall into an impalpable Powder in great Measure;) be taken three Times every Day, Morning, Afternoon, and at Bed-time, in three or four Spoonfuls of Water, Small-Beer, Wine, or Wine and Water; drinking after each Dose the third Part of the following Decoction:

Take two Ounces, two and half, or three, of Alicant Soap; slice it thin, and dissolve it in a Quantity of Water sufficient to make a Pint and half of the Decoction. Strain it, and sweeten it with Honey, or Sugar, to the Taste.—*The Lady's Companion*, 1751.

4

Some Afflictions of the Lower Bowel and Suggestions for their Relief

The regular action of the functions of the Rectum are so important to the health and the enjoyment of life, that I regret the diseases to which this organ is so commonly liable, and which are so painful and distressing to bear, should not have received more attention from the profession; particularly when I consider that the female sex are such frequent sufferers from these complaints, and to whom, from the delicacy of the situation of these diseases, there appears an almost insurmountable obstacle to the attainment of the desired relief. This delicacy on the part of the patient, has, doubtless, been the chief cause of the feeling of indifference shown by medical practitioners towards these particular complaints, rather than the want of inclination to acquire the necessary information on the subject.—*Diseases of the Rectum and Anus*, 1851.

What are the causes of constipation? Of all the causes which originate and establish habitual constipation, there is undoubtedly none so common as inattention to the calls of Nature, which are too frequently not only ill-obeyed, but even set aside by every trivial circumstance. How often does it happen that a lady, finding it not quite convenient to retire to the cabinet at the moment she experiences an admonition, defers it to a more favourable opportunity, but this opportunity having arrived, her efforts are powerless, the bowels will not act, and she has perforce to abandon the effort, and retire from the contest disappointed and discomfited. It should be remembered that the evacuation of the bowels is a natural and necessary function, without which health cannot be enjoyed or preserved, and some resolution should consequently be exercised in order to promote this object. Some people never think of going to the closet unless urged by an imperative necessity which they cannot resist.

The want of proper conveniences has undoubtedly much to do with the prevalence of constipation. As a rule, little or no attention is paid to the situation and construction of the water-closet. It is either placed in some out-of-the-way corner, where no one can find it, or it is so prominently situated that it requires a vast amount of manœuvring to pay a visit without the fact being patent to every one in the house. Not uncommonly in the country it is a long way off, quite at the bottom of the garden, and very likely you have to walk right past the dining-room windows to get to it. Instead of being a bright, cheerful little chamber, where you might pass five or ten minutes with a certain amount of comfort, and moralise on things in general, it is a cold, damp, repulsive room which gives you the shivers even to look at.

In the construction of houses, too much attention cannot be given to determining the situation in which the water-closets are to be placed, in order that the access may be easy and the egress private. In many houses there is only one water-closet for the whole family. There should never be less than two, and it would be a good thing if one were reserved exclusively for ladies. People put themselves to a vast amount of expense in fitting up

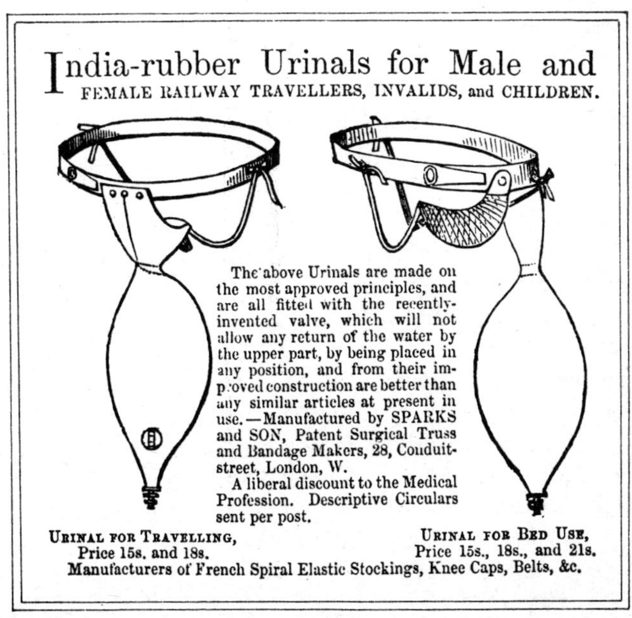

apartments and providing entertainment for their friends, but they too often neglect the one thing which is so essential for their comfort and well-being.—*The Family Physician*, 1883.

Thread-worms are of very common occurrence in children. They are little things looking just like a thread. They not unfrequently occur in immense numbers. They reside in quite the lower part of the bowel, from which circumstances they are often known as seat-worms. When only a few are present, they give rise to no inconvenience, and are usually only accidentally discovered in the stools. When they are numerous, they often cause itching or tickling of the back passage, which is sometimes very distressing, especially towards night.

A capital mode of treatment is to inject into the back passage a pint of cold water containing a table-spoonful of tincture of steel. This may be repeated once or twice a day until the worms have disappeared. An injection of infusion of quassia, or of salt and water, answers equally well. It is very desirable to pay attention to the general health, and steel wine, Parrish's Chemical Food, or cod-liver oil may be advantageously administered.

The patient should avoid touching the neighbourhood of the back passage, and should be scrupulously clean in person and clothing. The common Hindoo custom of washing after every act of defecation should be adopted. People suffering from worms should sleep alone. The food should be well cooked, and the hands should be thoroughly washed before and after every meal.—*Ibid*.

The mode of treatment of prolapsus recti I have not only found afford relief, but even effect a cure. In those cases however, where the base of the prolapsus is greatly constricted spasmodically, the fume of tobacco has been used. A common clay pipe answers every purpose, the small end being introduced into the rectum, whilst the bowl is filled with tobacco, which being ignited, is puffed with a bellows as often as it may be deemed necessary; pressure also being made round the verge of the anus, to prevent the escape of the smoke. No more than two or three puffs of smoke should be given at one time; and indeed, the greatest caution ought to be observed in the administration of this dangerous and uncertain remedy.—*Diseases of the Rectum and Anus*, 1851.

For a hypochondriacal person that is extremly tormented with winde; put a pair of bellows end into a clyster pipe; and, applying it into the fundament, open the bowels, so draw forth the winde.—*The Anatomy of Melancholy*, 1621.

I may mention that leeches, in attempts to apply them to the anus, may make their way into the rectum. A gentleman sent for me one evening, who complained of a very uneasy feeling in the rectum. He mentioned that he had endured considerable pain from an external pile, to which he had applied two leeches. The first, however, did not bite, but was lost, and subsequently could not be found. He had not the slightest idea that it was contained in the rectum (which I, however, suspected), and was greatly surprised when I told him that it was very probably the cause of his uneasiness. I recommended an injection of ox-gall, to which he consented, and the leech was soon discharged, almost dead, to his great astonishment and amusement.—*Diseases of the Rectum and Anus*, 1851.

If not for the edification, at least for the peculiar amusement of the reader, I will mention a few of the many cases where extra-ordinary substances have been extracted from the rectum. M. Nolet, surgeon to the King of France and Marine Hospital at Brest, relates the following curious case:—A monk wishing to get rid of a violent colic, introduced into the rectum a bottle of Hungary water, through the cork of which he had made a small opening to permit the fluid to flow into the intestine. In his anxiety to perform the operation well, he pushed the bottle so far that it completely entered into the gut. He could neither go to stool nor receive a lavement. A sage femme failed to insert her hand; the forceps and speculum were tried in vain; however, a boy, from eight to nine years of age, succeeded in introducing his hand and removed the bottle. M. Desault, in endeavouring to extract a porcelain jelly-pot of a conical form, and about three inches in length, which had been introduced for eight days, placed on two opposite points of its diameter two strong pincers, which, however, fractured it, so that he was compelled to extract the pieces in succession. M. Saucerotte withdrew a piece of wood three inches in length and two in width, with a corkscrew, which he inserted into the wood, while he steadied it with the fore finger of his left hand. M. Bruchman performed a similar operation with a gimlet.—*Ibid*.

The mischief which may be produced by too active purgation seems to have been well understood by the ancients; but the modern practitioner has too frequently rejected the advice which the sages of our profession have recorded for his instruction. 'He who takes a rough purge,' says Plutarch, 'to relieve his body from too great a load of food, may be compared to the Athenian, who finding the multitude of citizens troublesome to him, contrived to drive them out by filling the city with Scythians and wild Arabs.' I do not wish to invest the Grecian historian with the attributes of a medical oracle, but we may be allowed to borrow from him a figurative allusion to illustrate the importance of a precept which cannot be too frequently or too forcibly impressed upon the mind of the medical practitioner, who, I cannot but believe, is far too indiscriminate in this practice, the idea of purgation would seem to predominate over every other, he sweeps away the meconium of the new born child, and he administers a black dose to the expiring octogenarian.—*A Treatise on Diet*, 1837.

DR BUTLER'S PURGING ALE

Take polypody of the oak and senna, of each four ounces, of sarsaparilla two ounces, of aniseeds and carraway seeds of each an ounce, of scurvy grass half a bushel, of agrimony and maiden-hair of each a handful, beat all these easily and put them into a coarse canvas bag, and hang them in three gallons of ale, and in three days' time you may drink it.—*West Wickham Cookery Book*, 1934.

PLAIN HIERA-PICRA

Put one ounce of Hiera-Picra into one quart of brandy, let your bottle hold more than a quart that you may have room to shake it, let it stand five days near the fire, shaking it often and stop it close. This is a good purge. Take half a-quarter of a pint going to bed, drink a draught of warm ale or broth a little while afterwards. You may take it nine or ten days together. It opens the stomach, causes digestion, prevents green-sickness and kills worms in children.—*Ibid*.

5

Some Conditions of a Surgical Nature and Minor Problems of the Nose, Ears and Eyes

OF ULCERS

What we are to understand by the Word Ulcers, is a Solution of the soft Parts of our Bodies, together with the Skin, produced either by some internal Cause, or by Wounds and Contusions becoming inveterate.

Galen Defines an Ulcer to be an inveterate Erosion of the soft Parts, which prevents them from Consolidation; and it is observed that they arise from a Solution of Continuity, or a Destruction of the due Texture of the Parts, sometimes spontaneous, and at other Times arising from Wounds and Abscesses, either totally neglected, or ill managed. These Disorders may happen in any soft Parts of our Body, often internally, as in the Lungs, Liver, Palate, Fauces, Womb, Bladder, Bowels, etc., or axillary, as in the Parotid, the Exillary, Mamillary, Inguinal, and in all or any of the Glands, as also in the more soft Parts, as the Skin, Fat and Flesh, as in the Arms, Sides, Belly, Thighs, Legs and Anus: As for those arising from Wounds inflicted, Burns, Contusions and Abscesses, I think, as they differ in all Circumstances from real Ulcers, they ought not to be ranked in the same Class, because they are only the Effects of a former Cause; whereas Ulcers, properly Speaking, are Disorders sui Generis, and arise from some Indisposition of the Body, as from an Obstruction of the Menses, Dropsy, Lues Venerea, Small Pox, Evil, Cancer, Scurvy, Plague, and the like; and according to their Complexion and Malignity, they have taken their various Names. Thus if the Discharge is a Bloody Water, it is called, an Ichorous or Sanious Ulcer:

Viscid stinking Matter.	*Sordid or putrid.*
A thin Pus	*Purulent.*

With a Fungus	*Hypersarcosis.*
Lips hard and like Seams	*Callous.*
Hollow with Meanders	*Sinuous.*
When with knotted Veins, etc.	*Varicous.*
Obdurate and dry and of long Continuance	*Annual.*
A black Discharge, and the Bone bare	*Carious.*
There are also several Species in the West Indies	*Verminous.*

In our Attempts to cure any Species of these Ulcers, the first Step is to find out the internal Disease, that the Blood may be cleansed from such Impurities as produced it; and here we must call to our Air, the Pharmaceutic Part of Surgery, without which all topical Applications will not answer the Intent, but will be no more than if we should make an Effort to drain a Pond of Water, before the Springs which supply it are either stop'd up, or turn'd another Way; besides, if we should get such Ulcers to heal, it is dangerous on Account of the Humours being suppress'd and thrown back into the Mass of Blood, the consequence of which, like other Poisons, may in Time produce either an Asthma, an Epilepsy, a Vertigo, an Erysipelas, Blindness, and other terrible Disorders; but even if neither of these should fall out, the Patient's Life may be cut off suddenly. It has happened in robust Constitutions, that after the Ulcer has conglutinated, the Patient has become unhealthy, till such Time as that great Physician Nature has forced the Ulcer open again, or despumated and thrown off the noxious Humour by a kindly Diarrhœa.— *Practical Cases and Observations in Surgery,* 1751.

A Hackney-Coachman driving between London and Bristol, had the Misfortune, at Harehatch about 7 miles from Reading, to fall into a Quarrel with some officers of the Army; and after having beat and bruised two of them, a third, exasperated at the ill usage he saw his Companions meet with, stept up and barbarously made a thrust at the Coachman with a Hanger, which penetrated the Cavity of the Thorax in such a manner, that the Air discharged from the external Orifice of the Wound extinguished several Candles, when held near to it. Mr Smythers and I being called from Reading to the Patient's Assistance, we, upon a careful Inspection and Examination of the Wound, found its Direction oblique, and its Orifice small. Every Symptom pronounced him in imminent Danger, if not absolutely past all Hopes of Recovery; for he was afflicted with the most excruciating Pains, and laboured under an incredible Difficulty of breathing, attended with an almost uninterrupted Syncope, from which last Symptom, we concluded, that the Diaphragm must necessarily be hurt.

The first step we took was to dilate the Wound, in order to make its Orifice more depending; after which we dressed according to Art, and blooded the Patient copiously. We also ordered him to be kept very low, and his Intestines to be frequently emptied by Clysters of Broth. He had emollient Substances, such as Sperma Ceti, Oil of sweet Almonds, and others of a like Nature often exhibited with the pectoral Decoction. He was kept very low, and prohibited the use of meat of every kind. What he drank was of a soft, balsamic and mucilaginous Quantity. The Venesections were continued, as the Symptoms required, and were very frequent during the first two or three Days. However, dangerous as the Wound at first seemed to be, by persisting carefully in the above Method, a perfect Cure was obtained in a month, and the Patient still enjoys good Health and a vigorous Constitution.—*Ibid.*

A lad received a Blow or Kick from one of the Horses in a Cart, which fractured the frontal Bone on the left side, in several pieces, and bent the Forehead inwards, like to a large Bruise in a tin, copper, or pewter Vessel; the Depressure reached near down to the Minor Canthus: A neighbouring Quack-Surgeon, spiritually authorised, to lop, dismember, etc. was fetched in to the Boy's Assistance, who immediately promised a perfect Cure, and in a short time.—But after having him under his Care, for five or six days, dressing the Wounds, (I doubt not) but with his Samaritan Balsam, never failing Plaisters, and such like Nostrums; the Patient became raving, and was afflicted with convulsive Spasms.

On which the Boaster much affrighted, took his Leave, and pronounced him irrecoverable. Early in the Morning I was called out of my Bed to the Patient, when I found him delirious, with an Inflammation on his Head and Face of the Erysipalous Kind, and swoln to so great a degree that I could scarce discover either his Eyes, Nose, or Mouth; and the whole Head seemed a Mass of soft Dough. On removing the Pledgits, and extracting the Plugs cram'd into his Head, there flowed a bloody Ichor from the inside of the Cranium; the Wound was larger than a Crown-piece. On searching with my Probe, I found the Edges of the fractured Bones, forming an Arch, with part of the frontal and temporal Muscles lacerated.

Having every thing necessary for trepaning, I made an Incision in the superior part of the frontal Bone, first measuring with a String from the middle of the Chin to the coronal Suture, lest I should injure the Sinus Longitudinalis of the Dura Mater.— Having removed the Scalp and Pericranium, I cut out a piece of the sound Bone, with about a fifth of the Fracture, on which issued out some extravasated Blood; it was through this Perforation that the Elevator was introduced, between the Bone and Meninges of the Brain, and the deprest or inward bent Bones were raised up and restored to their natural Situation, whilst the loose Fragments were taken away.

During the Operation, Matter or Pus flowed from the inferior part of the Wound, and through the lacerated Dura Mater, which

Membrane I opened, and there discovered a Fragment or Splinter of the Bone, which had been forced through into the Brain. This I extracted, and then dilated the Membranes the whole extent of the Wounds, on which near half a common Glass full of the cortical Substance of the Brain and Pus were discharged; this opening was sufficient to prevent a second Suppuration, since the Discharge afterwards daily decreased, and the Cure was perfected in good Time; some of the Bones rejoined themselves, after they had scaled around their Edges; a low Diet, Bleeding, Blistering, Fomentation, etc., were carefully used during the whole Course of the Cure, which was at last happily finished to the great Satisfaction of his Parents and himself.—*Ibid.*

Bishop Berkeley speaks of tar water as being a cure for 'foulness of blood, ulceration of the bowels, consumptive coughs, pleurisy, pneumonia, erysipelas, asthma, indigestion, cachectic and hysteric cases, gravel, dropsy, and all inflammations.' In fact, about a century ago tar water was for a time regarded as universal panacea.

When the tar water mania was at its height, an ingenious hoax was perpetrated on the Royal Society. It appears that a sailor who had broken his leg was advised to communicate to that learned body a report of his case. The account he gave was that, having fallen from the top of the mast and fractured his leg, he had dressed it with nothing but tar and oakum, and yet in three days he was able to walk as well as before the accident. The story at first sight appeared quite incredible, as no such efficacious qualities were known in tar, and still less in oakum: nor was a poor sailor to be credited, on his own bare assertion, of so wonderful a cure. The Society very reasonably demanded a fuller relation, and the corroboration of the evidence. Many doubted whether the leg had been really broken. That part of the story had been amply verified. Still, it was difficult to believe that the man had made use of no other application than tar and oakum; and how *they* could cure a broken leg in three days, even if they could cure it at all, was a matter of the utmost wonder. Several letters passed between the Society and the patient, who persevered in the most solemn asseverations of having used no other remedies, and it appeared beyond a doubt that the man spoke the truth. But charming was the plain, honest simplicity of the sailor: in a postscript to his last letter he added the words: 'I forgot to tell

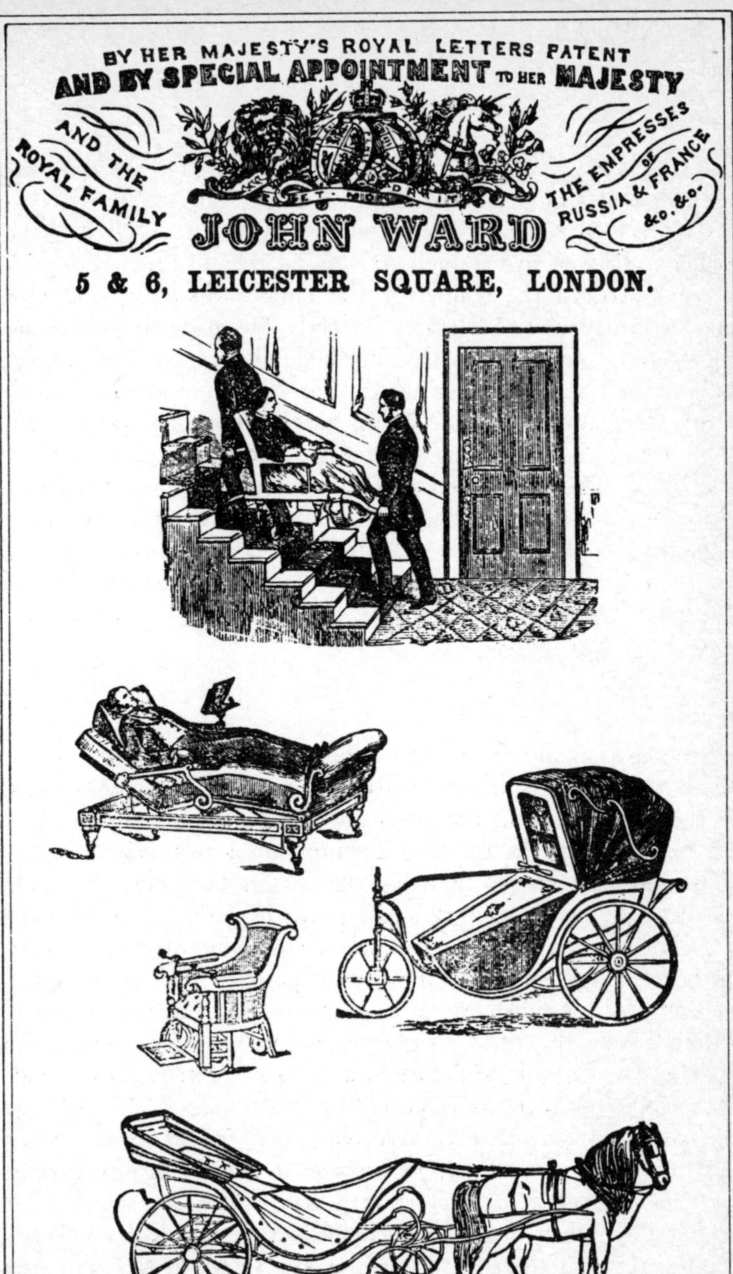

BY HER MAJESTY'S ROYAL LETTERS PATENT
AND BY SPECIAL APPOINTMENT TO HER MAJESTY
AND THE
ROYAL FAMILY
THE EMPRESSES OF RUSSIA & FRANCE
&c. &c.
JOHN WARD
5 & 6, LEICESTER SQUARE, LONDON.

your honours that the leg was a wooden one.'—*The Family Physician*, 1883.

It is reported that a specimen which remains one of the most valued in the Hunterian Museum cost Mr Hunter no less than £500 in 1783, namely, the skeleton of O'Brien, the Irish giant, seven feet seven inches high. It appears that O'Brien had heard of and dreaded the scalpel of the famous dissector, and took special precautions to frustrate his ends. He made an Irish league with several compatriots that his body should be taken to sea, and securely sunk in deep water; but Mr Hunter, more subtle than the giant, had made a big bargain with the undertaker, who arranged that during the funeral progress towards the sea the coffin should be locked up in a barn while its guardians were drinking at a tavern. The corpse was speedily extracted, and a sufficient weight of stones substituted; and Hunter soon rejoiced in the possession of his prize, which he drove to Earl's Court in his own carriage, and quickly converted into a skeleton.— *Eminent Doctors*, 1885.

To remove small articles from the nose, take a pair of small pliers and open them gently in the nostril without giving pain; at the same time, put the finger above the substance and press it downwards—not the finger and thumb so as to pinch the nose. If this does *not* answer, draw out the scissors and tickle the inside of the nose, or give a very small pinch of snuff, so as to make the child sneeze. In either the nose or ear, after stretching them open for a few minutes, it may be possible for you to get a bodkin past the substance, and so draw it out; but if you do not succeed, take the child to a surgeon, or you may inflame the place and make it ulcerate. Peas and beans are of more consequence than stones or metal substances, for they soon swell with the moisture and warmth of the place. I have myself known a pea left in the nostril of a poor neglected child till it began to sprout; fortunately by that time it had become so soft that it was easily broken down and removed, and the ulcer prevented coming through the side. In case of any insect getting into the ear, fill it with oil, and the insect will die immediately.—*Till the Doctor Comes*, 1870.

SALT & SON'S IMPROVED CLINICAL THERMOMETER.

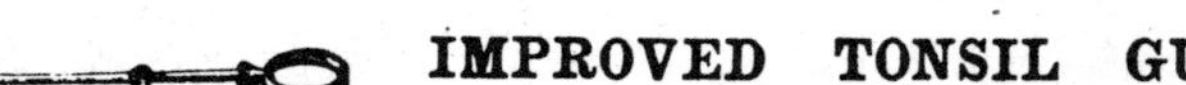

SCALE 2/3 SIZE

This Thermometer is fixed into an *aluminium* case, and is *propelled* and *retracted* in a manner somewhat similar to the American pencils—viz., by rotating the small end to the right or left respectively. In addition to being portable when sheathed and long when protruded, it was the first instrument in which *case and thermometer* are *inseparable*; and as, when retracted, the thermometer is wholly within the case, it is protected from being broken whilst the index is being replaced. The instrument is neat in appearance, and convenient for the waistcoat pocket or the ordinary dressing-case.—Price 16s. 2d., post-free.

INVENTORS AND PATENTEES,

SALT & SON, Birmingham, Surgical Instrument Manufacturers to the Hospitals.

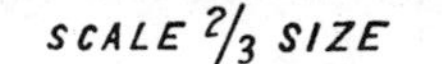

IMPROVED TONSIL GUILLOTINE.

By Mr. JOHN EWENS, of Cerne Abbas.

This instrument has metal guards passing from the two finger-rings to near the circular blade. Their use is to prevent the patient closing his mouth while the tonsil is being transfixed by the barbed spear, or during the excision of the tonsil, thus obviating the necessity of a separate gag, and rendering the operation less difficult.

HAWKSLEY'S STANDARD WEIGHING APPARATUS,

Suitable for the use of Physicians, Hospitals, Asylums, Prisons, Insurance Offices, Workhouses, and other Institutions. Price £5 5s. and £7 7s.

Inventor, Patentee, and Sole Maker, HAWKSLEY, 4, Blenheim-st., Bond-st., London, W.

In some cases considerable ingenuity is required to extract the foreign body from the ear. In one instance a small ivory ball had been detached from the top of a pen-holder in the care of a little boy. Syringing had done no good, and the forceps failed to grasp it and only pushed it in further. At last it was extracted by bringing the point of a small brush, dipped in glue, in contact with its surface, allowing the glue to harden, and then removing brush and ball together. This is a hint that might be of service in difficult cases.

The case is recorded of a nurse who, having failed to remove a button from a child's ear, actually *tried to push it out the other side*. We need hardly say that not only would such a thing be impossible but such treatment is highly dangerous.—*The Cyclopaedia of Practical Medicine*, 1833.

The treatment of deafness is not on the whole very satisfactory. In the first place the ears should be examined for wax by means of the speculum, and should there be an accumulation it must be removed by syringing as already directed. Should there be no wax the introduction of a drop or two of glycerine may do good. Should the general health be below par, iron and cod-liver oil may be given advantageously. Often benefit is derived from taking a table-spoonful of the tonic quinine mixture three or four times a day. For old people, or those who have done much brain-work, phosphorus, or the hypophosphites, may be employed with a fair chance of success, although of course they often fail to do any good.—*Ibid*.

Sir Hans Sloane's Receipt for Soreness, Weakness, and several other Distempers of the Eyes.
Take of prepared Tutty, one Ounce; of Lapis Haematites prepared, two Scruples; of the best Aloes prepared, twelve Grains; of prepared Pearl, four Grains. Put them into a Porphyry or Marble Mortar, and rub them with a Pestle of the same Stone very carefully, with a sufficient Quantity of Viper's Grease, or Fat, to make a Liniment; to be used daily, Morning or Evening, or both, according to the Conveniency of the Patient.

The Doctor prescribes Bleeding and Blistering in the Neck, and behind the Ears, in order to draw off the Humours from the Eyes; and afterwards, according to the Degree of the Inflammation, or Acrimony of the Juices, to make a Drain by Issues between the Shoulders, or perpetual Blister. And for washing the Eyes, recommends cold Spring-Water. And the best inward Medicines, which he has experienced, to be Conserve of Rosemary-Flowers; Anti-epileptic Powders, such as Pulvis ad Guttelam, Betony, Sage, Rosemary, Eyebright, wild Valerian Root, Castor, etc., washed down with a Tea made of the same Ingredients; as also Drops of Spirit Lavendulae composit, and Sal Volat. Oleos.

If the Inflammation returns, the Doctor says, drawing about six Ounces of Blood from the Temples by Leaches, or Cupping on the Shoulders, is very proper.

The Liniment is to be applied with a small Hair Pencil, the Eye winking, or a little opened.—*The Lady's Companion*, 1751.

Spectacles and Eye-glasses. We must say a word or two on this subject. The absolute necessity of purchasing the glasses under the direction of a qualified person, and of not going into a shop at random and taking just what the shopman gives you, has already been pointed out. In the mechanical arrangement of the lenses there are two or three points worthy of attention. The frames should be of metal, and sufficiently strong to prevent twisting or loss of weight. Steel is probably the best, although some people prefer gold. Lightness is, of course, essential to comfort. The nose piece, or saddle, should be carefully adjusted to fit the nose. Their pattern is a matter of taste, though the oval is generally considered to be the most becoming. The lenses themselves may be made of crystal—that is, Brazilian quartz—or of crown glass. The crystal is harder than glass, and is therefore less likely to scratch, and is not so liable to get broken. Moreover, it takes a higher polish, and being more refractive, it may be made of less thickness than glass. The great difficulty is to get a piece of crystal free from specks and impurities. Dishonest dealers often supply crown glass for crystal. The best way to distinguish between them is to apply a file to the edge of the material; glass cuts readily, but crystal is much harder. Crown glass lenses are very good, and may be used when the spectacles have to be changed often, or when expense is an object. Tinted or coloured lenses are sometimes used, but only when they are made of glass. As a rule, they are objectionable, because they remove the natural stimulus of white light, and thus make the retina unduly sensitive.

Eye-shades are sometimes used with advantage, especially when a bright light is objectionable. They may be made of fine fabric, of gauze coloured black, or, what is still better, plain grey. It is curious that shades are not more largely used as protectors for the eyes by artisans and others employed in work producing chips or fragments. Blue gauze wire set in a spectacle frame would answer the purpose admirably, especially if it were somewhat cup-shaped, so as to guard the eyes at the side. When the particles are not hard or are not driven with force, and especially when accurate light is required, as in lathe-work, thick glass set as spectacles would suffice. For reading, a shape that will protect the eyes from the direct rays of light is useful.—*The Cyclopaedia of Practical Medicine*, 1833.

6

Concerning the Diseases of Women and with Especial Reference to Methods of Examination

The practice of *man*-midwifery is one among the noxious weeds which the rank luxuriance of civilization has produced, and since its introduction it has thriven with unrestrained vitality and ever-increasing strength, until at length it spreads its Upas shadow far and wide over our land, and treacherously, mysteriously, and silently distils the poison of its presence deep into the sanctuaries of domestic life.

The first thing he always does, when he comes to the bed-side, is to make *an examination per vaginam!*' with other observations equally harrowing to the sensibilities of a husband.

What shock so terrible to a man who, rejoicing in the delightful sentiment of a wife's purity, discovers that all he held dearest and most sacred, all which he would shield from profanation with the last drop of his life's blood, has been invaded by the presence, and *violated by the actual contact* of the *man*-midwife? The doctor may be a sober, discreet, oily man, of staid appearance, and a very pattern of propriety; or he may be a vulgar, low-bred person, in his leisure consorting with those of a similar bent; or

> 'Yonder a vile physician, blabbing
> The case of his patient . . . ;'

or he may be a tippling, jovial fellow, who at some roystering party is always called on for 'a good song,' sure to have as its theme wine, love and woman,—for accoucheurs are mortals like other men; or he may be some tyro in 'the art,' just let loose from his course of. walking the hospitals, strong in syphilitic cases, and with all the recollections of a young person's life fresh upon him; nevertheless, whatever he be, *the very inmost secrets of your wife's person* are known to him, the veil of modesty has been rudely torn aside, and the sanctity of marriage exists but in the name.

If the reader views with disgust and horror the above rules of ordinary practice in *man*-midwifery—and what man is base enough (save an accoucheur) not so to regard them?—these feelings will be intensified a thousand-fold by the contemplation of the latest invention of 'obstetric art.' We allude to the SPECULUM. The adoption of this instrument, as we are informed, is now becoming general; and its employment plunges its wretched victim, woman, down into the lowest depth of infamy and degradation. We will not pollute our pages by describing its method of action; suffice it to say, that, to the sense of *touch*, common to all midwifery practice, is added, in its application, that of *sight*; exposure the most complete of all which modesty, even in the most abject of races, invariably conceals.—*Hints to Husbands*, 1857.

Touching, as it is commonly called, is the Introduction of a Finger up the Vagina, as far as the Os Uteri, to find the Condition it is in, the State of the Membranes, and what Part of the Child presents.

How the Patient is to be placed while the Operator is touching her, is not very material; but how she ought to be placed during her Delivery, is a Point not altogether determined, some being for doing it standing; others, sitting on the Stool, or the Knee of some of the Females in Waiting; whilst others are for delivering the Woman lying in or upon the Bed; and these also differ in their Opinions, whether the Woman should lie on her Back, or on one Side. I shall offer my Reasons for the Position, which I have found by Experience to be the best, safest, and easiest for the Patient, as well as most convenient for the Operator: But I must premise to the Reader, that I am here speaking of natural Births only; in preter-natural or difficult Births, indeed, the Position of the Woman must, in some Particulars, be varied according to the Case; but in general, in those Cases too, the Posture here laid down is best.

A Tradesman's Wife fell into Labour at the usual Time. She had a slow, tedious, but safe Delivery; was some Hours upon the Stool, with the Midwife attempting to deliver her at every Pain, which were but slow; at last, however, she brought forth a living Child, which the Midwife gave to a Bystander, as soon as she could get the Navel-string tied and cut; and then she brought away the After-birth, after which followed the Blood that was extravasated; and tho' the Midwife put the Patient to Bed with

the usual Care and Expedition, yet the Cold she got had like to have killed her; for the Lochia were checked, and an Inflammation of the Womb ensued, which, with much Difficulty, I at last removed. Many repeated Instances of the like Kind I can give, both of some Peoples dying for Want of immediate Help, and of others being very near it, although they had timely Assistance; all of which were delivered upon the Stool or Knee; and no other apparent Cause of the Obstruction could be found; which, indeed, is sufficient of itself; for immediately upon the Exit of the Child and Afterbirth, the cold external Air must rush into the Womb, the bad Consequences of which are very evident.

The Inconvenience to the Operator is also greater than when the Patient is lying; for no Person can bend the Elbow-joint to thrust or pull with the Strength upwards or downwards, as sideways. The same Inconveniences, both to the Patient and Operator, attend a Delivery, when standing, except that the Os Coccygis cannot be so pressed inwards, as when sitting.

Most of these Inconveniences are avoided by deliverying the Patient lying in or on the Bed, for the Woman will be less apt to swoon or faint away, or to catch Cold, because the Cloaths may be kept closer about her Thighs, and the Operator may perform his Part with more Ease, and in less Time, especially if the Patient lies on one Side: For, when a Woman lies on her Back, the Bedding must be pressed down by her Weight, which makes it more difficult for the Operator to turn the Child in the Womb, especially if it be necessary to introduce his Hand betwixt the Os Pubis and the Child; because the Bedding is higher where his Elbow is, than where the Woman's Buttocks are.—*An Essay Towards a Complete New System of Midwifery*, 1751.

NEW SYSTEM OF MIDWIFERY

A person having miscarried seven Times, as near as she could tell in the latter End of the third, or Beginning of the fourth Month, sent for me when she expected to miscarry, having the usual Complaints which had preceded and attended her former Abortions, and it being about the Time she was wont to miscarry: I asked all the necessary Questions but could get very little Satisfaction from either the Patient or Midwife, relating to the Foetus, or Secundines of former Abortions, but flattered myself there was no Scirrhus in the Womb, as she had not the usual concomitant Symptoms. As I found she must inevitably miscarry again, I ordered them to preserve whatever came from the Uterus, if the Abortion should happen during my Absence, and to let me know directly: It was accordingly preserved, and I found in it as sound a Foetus as well as could be perceived in that State; and there seemed also to be no Manner of Defect in the Secundines; wherefore I concluded the Cause must be in the Mother's Form or Constitution. She was a healthy, but not robust Woman; her Complexion rather pale and fair, than sanguine; and her Arteries were small, with a feeble Pulse, even in her best State of Health.

She soon recovered after this Abortion, when I desired her to let me know, whenever she suspected she was again pregnant, that I might try to prevent a Miscarriage; I then ordered a Medicine, composed of gentle Corroborants with Stomachics, which agreed very well with her, and she regained her lost Appetite and Strength. Some Time after this she sent for me, having not had her Menses at the usual Time; her Pulse was then feeble, and she had not the usual Uneasiness from the Obstruction, nor yet any Symptoms that usually attended the Eruption of the Menses; wherefore I only ordered her to continue in the Method as above, and watched her very diligently.

About a Week before the Time the Menses should appear again, she began to have Complaints that used to precede their Eruption; wherefore I ordered six Ounces of Blood only to be taken from the Arm, and gave her a gentle Opiate at Night; this I repeated in six Days, she still taking the Medicines as before. A Week before the third Month, I ordered about four or five Ounces more of Blood to be taken; and the third or fourth Day after, to take four Ounces more; and again on the fourth Day to be repeated; and each Night after Bleeding she took the Opiate; so that in about nine Days she only lost twelve or thirteen Ounces of Blood. The Week before the fourth Month, she lost four Ounces more from the Arm; she still continuing the Medicines as prescribed, till she entered the sixth Month of Pregnancy, without any other Bleeding; and then went on to her full Time, and brought forth a living Child. After the first Miscarriage, she had been blooded every Time she was pregnant; but then they took twelve Ounces at a Time, without considering that her feeble Pulse would not bear the Loss of such a Quantity, neither had they considered to open a Vein at the proper time.

When the Uterus is in too lax a State, occasioned by long and great Discharges of the Fluor Albus; from the Os Uteri being over-stretched, and kept a long Time distended in former Labours, or from any other Cause, it is evident, if any Pressure is made against the Os Uteri from within the Womb, it must yield thereto and open, and thereby permit the Ovum or Embryo to slip out.—*Ibid.*

A lady of rank, labouring under a severe menorrhagia, suffered with that irritable and unrelenting state of stomach which so commonly attends uterine affections, and to such a degree, that every kind of ailment and medicine was alike rejected. After the total failure of the usual expedients to procure relief, and the exhaustion of the resources of the regular practitioner, she applied to the celebrated Miss Prescott, and was *magnetized* by the mysterious spells of this modern Circe. She immediately, to the astonishment of all her friends, ate a beefsteak, with a plentiful accompaniment of strong ale; and she continued to repeat the meal every day, for six weeks, without the least inconvenience! But the disease itself, notwithstanding this treacherous amnesty of the stomach, continued with unabated violence, and shortly afterwards terminated her life.—*A Treatise on Diet*, 1837.

OF THE FUROR UTERINUS

Salacity in Women, attended with Impudence, Restlessness, and a Delirium, is called the Furor Uterinus. I should choose to refer this Disorder to the Head, as there is sometimes a Melancholy, and sometimes a maniacal Delirium. The Patients delight to talk obscenely, and sollicit Men to satisfy their Desires, both by Words and Gestures.

It arises from a too great Sensibility, or Inflammation of the Pudenda, or Parts wherein the venereal Stimulus resides, which are chiefly the Clitoris and Vagina; or the too great Abundance and Acrimony of the Fluids of those Parts; or both these Causes may exist together.

In the Delirium Maniacum, the Patient is intirely shameless;

in the Melancholicum more reserved, and her Folly is confined to fewer Objects.

It may proceed from the Abuse of hot Aperitives; thus Sal Ammoniac, Borax, and Cantharides have produced it; from powerful Emmenagogues in hot and bilious Constitutions; sometimes from difficult and suppressed Menses; from Remedies given against Sterility. Musk dissolved in Oleum Aromaticum, and rubbed on the Membrum virile, has raised a Phlogosis in the Vagina, whence a Furor Uterinus ensued.

It is difficult of Cure in those whose Menses are difficult at first; in inveterate Cases; in old Subjects. It is easier cured, when the Furor Uterinus is essential, and the Delirium symptomatic, than when the Delirium is essential, and the Furor symptomatic. The Maniacal Delirium is harder to manage than the Melancholic. If it continues a Month or two, the Fault of the Brain becomes obstinate, for it degenerates into real Madness.

The Indications of Cure are to diminish the Heat and Sensibility of the affected Parts. To cool, sweeten, and dilute the Blood, and to render it balsamic; or to pursue both Intentions at once.

The first Indication is answered by frequent and copious Bleedings, as in an incipient Madness; even to eight Times in two Days, if nothing forbids; if she faints, there is no Danger. She must likewise be purged, as mad Folks are, with Salap, Scammony, Diagrid. The Dose must be increased on third, as being hard to purge. Emetics are also good, for they evacuate the Bile, which abates the Acrimony of the Humours.

In a Delirium Melancholicum (lawful) Coition may be admitted, for I knew a Woman of some Consequence run to the Guard-Room, and return perfectly cured.—*The General Practice of Physic*, 1763.

The Solitary Vice. Terrible as are the bodily diseases and moral ruin which result from the Social Vice, it may be questioned whether the infirmity and degradation of the human race from the 'Solitary Vice' is not the greatest of the two evils. Habits of self-pollution, which attracted the attention of philanthropists in the early days of Health Reform, and elicited the instructive writings of Graham, Alcott, the Fowlers and others, are still more prevalent now. The only remedy for this evil, as well as for that of prostitution, lies in a health education of the people in the broadest acceptation of the term.

The manner in which the great majority of American children are fed, if it does not ruin their digestive organs and render them dyspeptics or consumptives, is sure to produce permanent congestion, with constant irritation in the pelvic viscera, resulting in a precocious development and morbid intensity of amativeness. Tea, coffee, flesh meats, to say nothing of the abominations of the baker and confectioner, are sufficient to account for the early tendency to sexual dissipation and debauchery manifested by a large portion of the children in our primary schools. Many a parent, now confiding in the purity and safety of his own son or daughter, might be appalled if he should investigate this subject. —*Sexual Physiology*, 1866.

The Theory of Sixt. Several years ago a work in manuscript was submitted to me for examination entitled 'An Exposition of the Mysteries of Nature concerning the Generation of Man and the Voluntary Choice of the Sex of the Progeny.' The author was P. F. Sixt, M. D., a practising Physician at Erfurt, Germany. After a critical examination of the reasoning and the facts, I became convinced that the theory advanced was in the main correct, and after submitting it to the test of direct experiment in several instances—all of which resulted in a confirmation of the theory—I purchased the work and published it.

Briefly stated, the theory advanced by Sixt is this: 'The organs of the right side, respectively, of the male and female, pertain to the male sex, and the organs of the left side to the female sex. In other words, the right testicle produces male "sperm-cells" and the right ovary produces female "sperm-cells" while the left testicle produces female "sperm-cells" and the left ovary female "germ-cells." The semen of the right testicle can not impregnate the ovum of the left ovary, nor can the ovum of the right ovary be impregnated with the semen of the left testicle. In order to have coition fruitful, the secretion of the right testicle must come in contact with the ovum of the right ovary, or the secretion of the left testicle must meet with the ovum of the left ovary.'

This theory is sufficiently plausible in its statement; and it has a tangible basis—anatomy itself. But its truth or fallacy can only be demonstrated by actual experiment. It was the opinion of Hippocrates that each testicle furnished its peculiar sperm; and others have held that the seed of the one testicle served to fructify the male, and that of the other the female eggs. But, so far as I can discover, Sixt was the first to advance the theory that each ovary contains its peculiar eggs, the right one the male, and the left the female ones. And I am inclined to think, from the result of certain experiments which some of my friends have made at my request, that, if there is any error in the theory of Sixt, it is in relation to the testicles, and not in relation to the ovaries; in other words, if the law of sex resides in either the male or female organs, and not in both, those organs are the ovaries.

According to the theory of Sixt, it is only necessary that the right or left testicle be firmly compressed or drawn up toward the abdomen, in the act of seminal emission, to beget a boy or a girl. It is always the case that, during coition, one or the other is drawn up so as to compress the spermatic vesicles; and, although the co-equal compression of the spermatic vessels of both sides from a drawing up of both testicles may be admitted as a possibility, yet there are many facts which seem to prove that emission is, ordinarily and normally, only from one side at one coition. Sixt gives certain rules as to bodily position in the act of sexual intercourse calculated to favor the compression of the organs of one or the other side as may be desired, and, although they would doubtless be sufficient with some persons, I do not deem them to be generally reliable, and therefore do not repeat them.—*Ibid.*

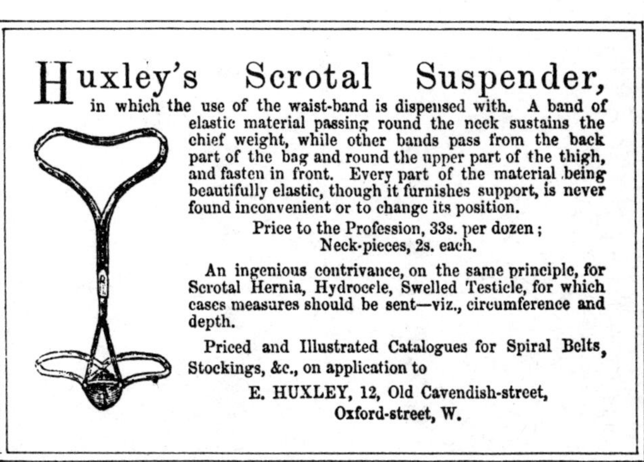

It is a fact, that if the body, and more particularly the brain, of any animal during the instant of procreation be exactly on a line

with the north and south poles, in ninety-nine cases in every hundred conception *will not* take place, but if it should, that the offspring will be deformed and very probably a hermaphrodite. And if the body and brain of the female be exactly east and west, with the head lying directly west, the progeny will be male; partaking equally of the characters and bodily configurations of both parents, but in a higher degree or more improved form, or in other words, the progeny will be more perfect, bodily and mentally, than the parents, provided they are in sound health.

But if the body of the mother, or even the head, be turned to either side, say for instance a northwest direction, the character of the progeny will be spirited, wild and unruly, and will partake more of the character, and in features more closely resemble, the father; but if the body and brain of the mother be in a southwest direction, the offspring will resemble the mother, and will be tame, gentle and quiet.

Now, if the body, etc., of the mother is on a direct line east and west, and the head lying east, the offspring will be of the female sex, and will be an improvement on the characters and the bodily organizations of both parents. If lying in a northeast direction, the offspring will resemble the father; and if in a southeast direction, more generally the mother. I have drawn a diagram, by referring to which you can more fully understand it.

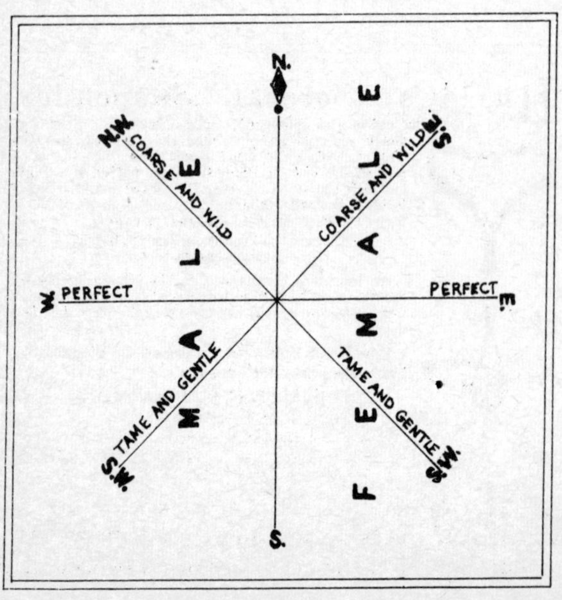

This is the whole secret. I shall make no comments on it, further than to say that it really seems to me to be plausible, but I am not well enough acquainted with physiology and magnetism to account for it on physiological principles, if it be a fact; but I suppose you will be able to decide immediately whether it be true or false. I await your answer with impatience.—*Ibid.*

7

In which are discussed the Care of Teeth and Treatment of their Diseases

If 40 Germans, at the age of 40, were compared with the same number of English, at the same age—all taken indiscriminately from the streets of Vienna and London—what would be the comparative number of sound teeth in the heads of the two classes? I shall attempt a calculation presently; mean time, it will be admitted on all hands, that the Germans are woefully afflicted with unsound teeth. What is the reason? A pair of mill-stones will grind only a certain quantity of corn—or last only a certain number of years. It is the same with the human mill-stones, or molares. They will only grind a certain quantity of food, or do a certain amount of labour, before they are worn out, like their namesakes in the mill. Now if the Germans eat one-third more than the English—and I firmly believe they do— then their teeth have one-third more of work, and ought to experience a corresponding degree of wear and tear. This, however, will not account for the premature decay of the teeth, but only for their wearing out sooner than under other circumstances. We must seek deeper for the causes. As the millstones are spoiled and rendered useless by allowing improper things to be mixed with the grain, as pebbles, etc. so the teeth are injured by the quality as well as by the quantity of our food. The oils, acids, tobacco, and other deleterious substances, for ever mixing with continental meals, must greatly injure the organs of mastication as well as of digestion.—*Pilgrimages to the Spas*, 1841.

As the Rheumatism appears in temperate, and a sudden Change of Weather; so it is with the Tooth-Ach, especially when the Weather is hot and cold by Fits.

The whole Intention of Cure consists in deriving and diverting the impure scorbutic Serum from the Head, and then carrying

it off through proper Emunctories; and afterwards in strengthen-
ing the Parts.

This is to be done by saline, emollient, purgative, Clysters;
by warm Pediluvia of Rain Water and Wheat Bran, with Venice
Soap, and used just before Bed-time; by Laxatives of Manna and
Cassia dissolved in Whey or Asses-Milk or mineral Waters. If
the Patient is plethoric or full of Blood, Bleeding in the Foot
will derive the Humours from the Head.

Outwardly may be applied Bags, filled with paragoric and
emollient Species, such as Elder, Melilot, and Camomile
Flowers, Bay and Juniper-Berries, Carraway and Millet Seeds,
and decrepitated Salt. They must be laid on warm, and are very
safe.

A Drop or two of Oil of Cloves, or Box, applied to a carious
Tooth with Cotton, are Medicines not to be despised. Camphor-
ated Spirit of Wine mixed with Saffron, Caster, and Opium,
made into a Liniment, and laid to the Gums and hollow Teeth,
often gives the Patient Ease.

When the Tooth-Ach proceeds from a rotten, hollow Tooth,
it will be best to burn the little nervous Cord, which is the Seat
of the Pain, with an actual Cautery; and then the Cavity may be
filled up with a Mixture of Wax and Mastich. I have known this
attended with great Success.

If this cannot, or is not permitted to be done, the only Remedy
left is to have the Tooth drawn.

It is now become a Practice, especially in France, upon drawing
a sound Tooth, to replace it in its Socket; where, with proper
Precautions, it will fasten again. Musgrave is the first that I
know of, who recommends this Practice. After the Extraction of
the Tooth, he advises a Gargle of Honey, mixed with the Juice of
the Herb Mercury, common Salt, and Spring-Water, and then to
put it in its former Place; and adds it will become more useful
than before.

The French Operators have improved this Hint; and when the
Tooth is rotten, or otherwise unfit to be replaced, they put
another sound human Tooth in the Room of it, when it can be
had; otherwise one of any other Animal, that is of a Size suitable
for the purpose.—*The General Practice of Physic*, 1763.

Creasote is a substance obtained by the distillation of wood tar.
It is an almost colourless liquid, having a powerful characteristic

odour. It is a favourite remedy for the *toothache*, and when a few drops are introduced into the hollow of a decayed and painful molar, it will usually afford relief.—*The Family Physician*, 1883.

The yellow threads in the middle of the red roses especially being powdered and drunk in the distilled water of quinces doth wonderfully stay and helpe the defluxions of rheume upon the gummes and teeth, and preventeth them from corruption, and fasteneth them that being loose, if they be washed and gargled therewith, and some vinegar of squilles added thereto.—*Theatrum Botanicum*, 1640.

An admirable Powder for the Teeth; by Dr Bracken, of Preston in Lancashire. Get Tartar of Vitriol, two Drams; best Dragons-Blood and Myrrh, of each half a Dram; Gumlac one Dram; of Ambergrease four Grains; and those that like it may add two Grains of Musk; mix them well, and make a Powder to be kept in a Phial close stopp'd.

The Method of using it is thus; put a little of the Powder upon a Saucer, or a Piece of white Paper; then take a clean Linnen Cloth upon the End of your Finger, just moisten it in Water, and dip it in the Powder, and rub your Teeth well once a Day if they be foul, washing your Teeth after with warm Wine or Water; if you want to preserve their Beauty only, twice a Week will be sufficient for its Use.—*The Lady's Companion*, 1751.

Water for Scurvy in the Gums. Take two quarts of spring water and one pound of right Flower-de-Luce root, and a quarter of a pound of rock alum, two ounces of cloves, two handfuls of red rose leaves, two handfuls of woodbine leaves, two ounces of columbine leaves, two handfuls of brown sage, and one of Rosemary, eight Seville oranges, peel and all, only take out the seeds, set these over the fire and let them boil a quart away, then take it off and strain it and set it over the fire again and put to it three quarts of claret and a pint of honey, let them boil half-an-hour, scum it well and when 'tis cold, bottle it for use; wash and gargle your mouth with it two or three times a day.—*West Wickham Cookery Book*, 1934.

8

Some Considerations of the Aliments, both Liquid and Solid

If we go to dine with a very rich man, or a city company, or other public body who constitute themselves the guardians of old English hospitality, what do we get to eat? If it is in the winter or autumn we may begin with six oysters, which are almost entirely composed of albuminates; then perhaps comes the turtle soup, which chemically is a pleasant decoction of albumen and gelatine, and it is remarkable that a gourmand who would discharge his cook for leaving a few drops of fat upon the surface of any ordinary soup, takes with his turtle huge quivering lumps of green and yellow fat, such as only the educated palate can tolerate and the strongest stomachs manage to digest, even with the help of cold punch and cayenne pepper. It is probable that in these first two courses sufficient nitrogen has been served to satisfy the requirements of the system; but see what follows, turbot and lobster sauce very likely, which again is almost purely albuminate. Then come the entrées, which are perhaps three in number, and consist (we quote from an actual *menu*) of *crême de volaille aux truffes*, or, in other words, purée of chicken with truffles; mutton cutlets, with which one may or may not get a potato; and *chaud-froid de caille*, which consists of cold quails encased in cold meat jelly. Here again, then, in the entrées we are confronted with the almost exclusive use of the albuminates. Next, we proceed to the joint, which is a slice of pure roast meat, and with it one gets, for a certainty, some potato and green vegetable, and perhaps some salad. Then will follow a bird of some kind—grouse, partridge, pheasant, wild duck, guinea fowl, according to season, or perhaps some greater delicacy, such as quail, or ortolan. With many of these birds it is considered little short of sinful to eat any vegetable, and with others there is served, at most, a few bread raspings, or a little bread sauce. Then come the sweets; and it is remarkable that even these are composed very largely of gelatine, and at most houses one finds the jellies in the ascendancy when compared with the sweets composed mainly of starchy matter and fruit. Cheese in some form brings the typical English banquet to a close. If reference be made to the standard diet, it will be seen that the albuminates should form one-fifth part of the total food, but in the *menu* we have supposed, and which is scarcely exaggerated, it will be observed that the albuminates constitute the major part of the dinner. This is of course quite wrong, and it is not to be wondered at that those misguided possessors of wealth who indulge almost daily in repasts of this kind should suffer from gout, dyspepsia, and derangements of the liver, and be compelled to fly to Homburg, or Carlsbad, or Buxton, Cheltenham, or Bath, to try the experiment of undoing that which has been brought about by gluttony, or ignorance, or both.—*The Family Physician,* 1883.

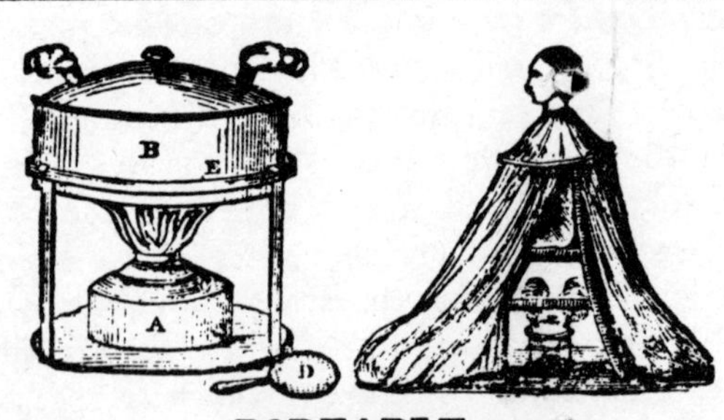

The influence of temperature on the process of digestion is remarkably shown in some of Dr Beaumont's experiments; he found that the gastric juice had scarcely any influence on the food submitted to it when the bottle was exposed to the cold air, instead of being kept at a temperature of 100°. He observed

on one occasion, that the injection of a single gill of water at 50°
sufficed to lower its temperature upwards of 30°; and that its
natural heat was not restored for more than half an hour. Hence
the practice of eating ice after dinner, or even of drinking largely
of cold fluids, is very prejudicial to digestion.—*The Family
Physician*, 1883.

The question often arises whether tea should be taken in the
early morning before getting up. The answer depends upon
whether it interferes with the appetite for breakfast or not.
The stimulating properties of tea make some people feel that
they do not want breakfast, and the result is they start the
day's work with an empty stomach, and, consequently, an
enfeebled body, and the habit of early tea-drinking is undoubtedly
injurious to them. Taken as a preliminary to active exercise
before breakfast, it is probably beneficial, and prevents undue
fatigue.

Alcoholic Drinks. In estimating the advantages and evils of
alcoholic fluids too much stress is usually laid on the properties
of alcohol and too little notice taken of the other constituents,
and the effects which they produce. Taken in moderate quantities
alcohol is a food, being utilised itself and sparing the other
constituents of our daily diet. It stimulates the heart and nervous
system, dilates the capillaries, giving a sensation of warmth to
the body, and aids digestion by promoting the secretion of the
digestive fluids. Probably its most valuable property is that men
like it, and it proves a pleasant adjunct to a meal. Theoretically,
a healthy man leading a healthy life requires no alcohol, and
the young are certainly better without it under ordinary circumstances; but practically, under modern conditions of life, few
men are injured by consuming a small amount of alcohol, and
the majority are distinctly benefited by it.

  Alcohol should only be taken at meal-time. Taken between
meals it is a poison irritating the digestive organs and preventing
them from responding to the calls of the system when food is
taken. The promiscuous brandy-and-soda, and the glass of port
wine taken between breakfast and lunch, cannot be too strongly
condemned.—*Gardener's Household Medicine and Sick Room Guide*,
1898.

One of the ill effects produced by an unsalted diet is the generation of worms. Mr Marshall has published the case of a lady who had a natural antipathy to salt, and was in consequence most dreadfully infested with worms during the whole of her life. In Ireland, where, from the bad quality of the food, the lower classes are greatly infested with worms, a draught of salt and water is a popular and efficacious anthelmintic. Lord Somerville, in his Address to the Board of Agriculture, gave an interesting account of the effects of a punishment which formerly existed in Holland. 'The ancient laws of the country ordained men to be kept on bread alone, *unmixed with salt*, as the severest punishment that could be inflicted upon them in their moist climate. The effect was horrible; these wretched criminals are said to have been devoured by worms engendered in their own stomachs.'— *Dr Paris on Diet and Regimen*, 1837.

9

Matters of Public Health and Sanitary Hygiene

Good people all! have a care of your skin,
Both that without and that within;
To the first give plenty of water and soap,
To the last little else beside water, we'll hope.

But always be very particular where
You get your water, your food, and your air;
For if these be tainted, or rendered impure,
It will have its effect on your blood—be sure.

The food which will ever for you be the best,
Is that you like most and can soonest digest;
All unripe fruit, and decaying flesh
Beware of—and fish that is not very fresh.

Your water, transparent and pure as you think it,
Had better be filtered and boiled ere you drink it;
Unless you know surely that nothing unsound
Can have got to it over or under the ground.

But of all things the most I would have you beware
Of breathing the poison of once-breathed air;
When in bed, whether out or at home you may be,
Always open your windows and let it go free.

With clothing and exercise keep yourself warm,
And change your clothes quickly if drenched in a storm;
For a cold caught by chilling the outside skin
Flies at once to the delicate lining within.

All you who thus kindly take care of your skin,
And attend to its wants without and within,

Need never of cholera feel any fears,
And your skin may last you a hundred years.

Notes on Nursing

OF THE FLUIDS WHICH PROCEED FROM THE BLOOD

Thus in every Season of the Year, when Perspiration is suppressed, Diseases are generated; hence in the Spring proceed Madness, Haemorrhages, Epilepsies, Quinsies, Gout, Rheums, Coughs, Lippitudes, Abscesses, Pustules, Rheumatisms, the Small-pox, Measles, catarrhal and continual Fevers. For when the Atmosphere is unequal and changeable, that is, sometimes moist, sometimes hot, sometimes cold, and sometimes windy, as in March, Diseases are generally rife. Then the Air becomes warm from putrid Moisture, which has long stagnated in the Earth, and the corruptible Exhalations begin to be dissolved, so that it is dangerous to be abroad, and to continue long in this Kind of Air, especially if the Body be weak.

Even the Diseases which happen in Summer, such as ardent, bilious, continual and intermitting Fevers, are not so much owing to Heat and Dryness, as to a cold moist Air, which predominates early in the Morning and in the Evening.

The Autumn, according to the Experience of all skilful physicians, is full of Diseases, on account of the Inequality and sudden Changes of the Weather.

The Diseases which reign in the Winter are certainly owing to intense Cold; hence Pleurisies and Peripneumonies, Rheumatisms, Defluxions, Gouts, acute Pains and Diseases of the Head. However, dry, serene, pure cold Weather increases the Spring of the Fibres, and strengthens the Body, if well cloathed, gives a proper Tone to, and invigorates all the Parts.—*The General Practice of Physic*, 1763.

Aerophobia. From one end of Germany to the other, among all ages, ranks, and professions, an AEROPHOBIA, or dread of fresh air, universally prevails! If you take a seat in the diligence or eilwagen, your German neighbour in the corner closes the windows immediately, lest a breath of pure air should enter the vehicle. On arriving at the hotel, half poisoned by the disoxygenated atmosphere of the coach, and enter your chamber, you find all the windows securely fastened, and the air of the apartment a mass of heavy mephitic vapour, like that which issues from a long unopened tomb. If you descend to the spies-saal, where the air is still farther vitiated by the fumes of tobacco, and throw open a window, you are stared at by the ober-kellner, the under-kellner, and every *gast* in the *haus*, as a person deranged. I had long puzzled my brains to account for this aerophobic phenomenon, and, at last, traced its cause to the German stove— that black brewery of mephitism, which, bearing a mortal antipathy to the fresh air of Heaven, imbues every one who sits near it with the same prejudice. In fine, the German exhibits as great a horror of oxygen, as he does a mania for azote!

And what is the consequence of this?—Why, that the Germans are ten times more susceptible of colds, rheumatism, face-aches, and tooth-aches, than the English, who live in a far more variable, wet, and ungenial climate. This aerophobia is one of the causes too, of that sallow, unhealthy aspect which all Germans, who are not forced to be much in the open air, exhibit. It is no wonder that they swarm like locusts round their numberless spas, in the Summer, to wash away some of those peccant humours engendered by their diet, and fermented by their stoves.—*Pilgrimages to the Spas*, 1841.

'Private Houses ought to be perflated once a Day, by opening Doors and Windows, to blow off the Animal Steams.'

'Houses, for the sake of Warmth fenc'd from Wind, and where the Carpenter's Work is so nice as to exclude all outward Air, are not the most wholsom.'

People who pass most of their Time in Air tainted with Steams of Animals, Fire and Candles, are often affected with nervous Distempers. Living constantly in Air that kills Vegetables, cannot be wholsom for animals.—*The Effects of Air on Human Bodies*, 1733.

Happily cases of acute poisoning from foul air are infinitely rare, but cases of slow poisoning from the same cause are, we fear, by far too common, both in the ill-constructed and unventilated dwellings of the poor, and in over-crowded workshops, work-houses, school-rooms, ball-rooms, churches, and theatres.

There are few things more astonishing than the poisonous misery to which the world of fashion submits, night after night, during the London season. A fashionable entertainment—a regular 'London crush'—almost recalls the piteous story told by Mr Holwell. Five or six hundred people jammed into a room calculated to contain perhaps a tenth part of them, and probably as many wax-lights as there are guests using up the oxygen, and adding their quota of carbonic acid to the already over-charged atmosphere. Is it surprising that windows stream with water, and the guests drip with perspiration, and in the very height of this misery fly for relief to those poisonous compounds called champagne? Is it to be wondered at, also, that scented soaps and perfumes scarcely suffice to mask the odour of organic effluvia; or that those who habitually participate in these delusive joys are among the most regular of the doctor's patients? Why it is that we so persistently turn night into day, and prefer to take our pleasure, not only in crowds, but after dark, when the air of our rooms is fouled by the combustion of gas and candles, is certainly a most inscrutable thing.—*The Family Physician*, 1883.

The very first care of nursing, the first and the last thing upon which a nurse's attention must be fixed, the first essential to the patient, without which all the rest you can do for him is as nothing, with which I had almost said you may leave all the rest alone, is this: *to keep the air he breathes as pure as the external air without chilling him*. Yet what is so little attended to? Even where it is thought of at all, the most extraordinary misconceptions reign about it. Even in admitting air into the patient's room or ward, few people ever think where that air comes from. It may come from a corridor into which all other wards are ventilated; from a hall, always unaired, full of the fumes of gas, dinners, of various kinds of mustiness from an underground kitchen, sink, wash-house, water-closet, or, even as I myself have had sorrowful experience, from open sewers loaded with filth; and with this the patient's room or ward is aired, as it is called—poisoned, it should rather be said. Always air from the air without, and that too from those windows through which the air comes freshest! From a closed court, especially if the wind does not blow that way, air may come as stagnant as from any air in corridor.—*Ibid.*

Housing. In selecting a house which is to be our home we should bear in mind how much the future happiness of the household depends on the house being healthy. No wealth or success can compensate for the worry and unhappiness caused by constant ill-health. With regard to the site for a house, Dr Parkes gives the following table stating the relative healthiness of the various forms of soil.

1. Rock
2. Gravel
3. Sandstone
4. Limestone
5. Sandy
6. Clay
7. Marshy

—*Gardener's Household Medicine*, 1898.

Communicated by a lady:

Mrs B, my Gibraltar friend, called yesterday, and told me all about her husband's illness, which was typhoid, as I expected. He was nearly at death's door. I give you part of our conversation.

Mrs A: Did you find anything wrong with the house?

Mrs B (not understanding): Wrong with the house! Why, it's one of the nicest houses in Gibraltar.

Mrs A: Oh yes, but did you have the drainage inspected with a view to discovering the cause of the disease?

Mrs B: Oh no; you see we came away in such a hurry.

Mrs A: But you surely do not intend going back to it without having an inspection made and getting things put right?

Mrs B: Put right! Why, my dear Mrs A, there cannot be much wrong, for the drain is always bursting, then everything has to be carried away.

Mrs A: Bursting! What makes it burst?

Mrs B: Oh, because it can't get away! All the drainage is bad at Gibraltar.

Mrs A: But perhaps you have no drains at all; and it is a cesspool that bursts.

Mrs B: Oh no; we have a drain from the house which goes to the main sewer in the middle of the road, but it takes a sudden bend, where everything stops, then it all bursts up near the kitchen door. There really cannot be much wrong (she repeated this for the second time), for it busts about *once a month.*

This is a good illustration of unconscious ignorance.

The dear good lady wept over her husband's sufferings, and dwelt on the narrow escape she had had of widowhood, and laughed over the bursting of the drain, and would not allow her mind to dwell on the possibility of anything being wrong there.—*Dangers to Health*, 1883.

HOUSE WITH EVERY SANITARY ARRANGEMENT FAULTY

This plate is intended to shew at one glance the most common sanitary faults of ordinary houses. In subsequent plates each fault will, as a rule for the sake of clearness, be given singly, in order that it may be more easily understood.

A *Water-closet* in the centre of the house.

B *House drain* under floor of a room.

C *Waste-pipe of lavatory*—untrapped and passing into soil-pipe of w.c., thus allowing a direct channel for sewer-gas to be drawn by the fires LL into the house.

D *Over-flow pipe of bath* untrapped and passing into soil-pipe.

E *Waste-pipe of bath* untrapped and passing into soil-pipe.

F *Save-all tray* below taps untrapped and passing into soil-pipe.

G *Kitchen sink* untrapped and passing into soil-pipe.
To these might have been added a *housemaid's sink.*

H *Water-closet cistern* with overflow into soil-pipe of w.c., thus ventilating the drain into the roof, polluting the air of the house, and polluting the water in the cistern, which also forms the water supply of the house for drinking and washing.

J *Rain-water tank* under floor, with over-flow into drain.

K *Fall-pipe* conducting foul air from tank fouled by drain gas, and delivering it just below a window.

M *Drain under house* with uncemented joints leaking; also a defective junction of vertical soil-pipe with horizontal drain; the drain laid without proper fall.

—Ibid.

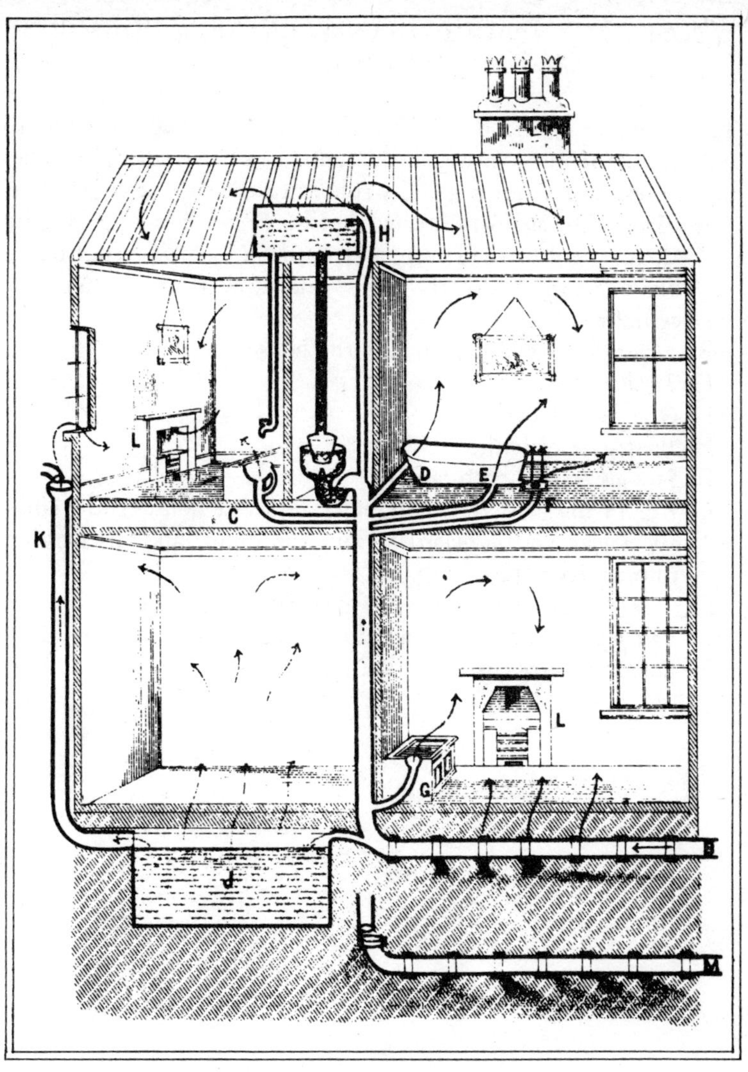

House with every sanitary arrangement faulty.

HOUSE WITH FAULTY SANITARY ARRANGEMENTS AVOIDED

This plate is intended to shew the reverse of the last, and to indicate the manner in which the faults can be rectified, but does not profess to lay down a strict rule as to the best arrangements.

A *Water-closet* against outer wall of house, with *soil-pipe* passing directly out of the house, and *ventilated* by a pipe continuing the soil-pipe above the eaves, and away from chimneys or windows.

BB *House drains* entirely outside the house.

C *Lavatory,*

D *Over-flow* of bath,

E *Waste-pipe* of bath,

F *Save-all tray* of bath, and

G *Kitchen sink*, to which might be added a housemaid's sink, all *trapped* and *disconnected* from the drain, and discharging into an open gully trap, L.

H *Over-flow* of cistern into the open air.

K *Fall-pipe* near bedroom window discharging into gully L.

M *Domestic cistern* distinct from w.c. cistern.

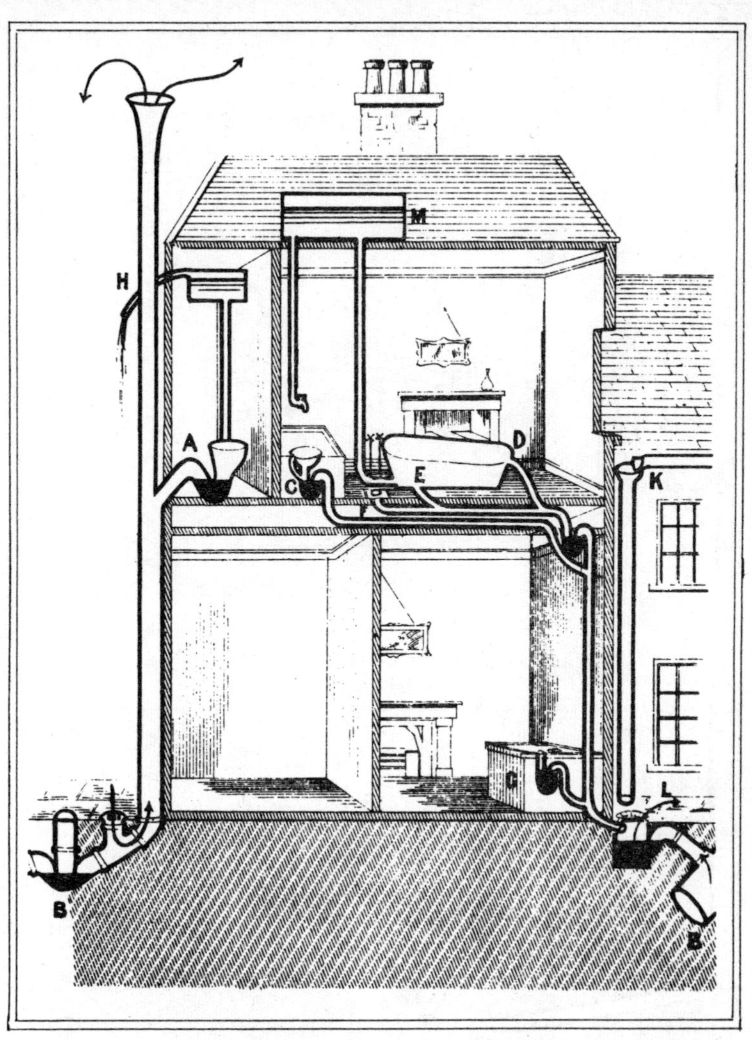

House with faulty arrangements avoided.

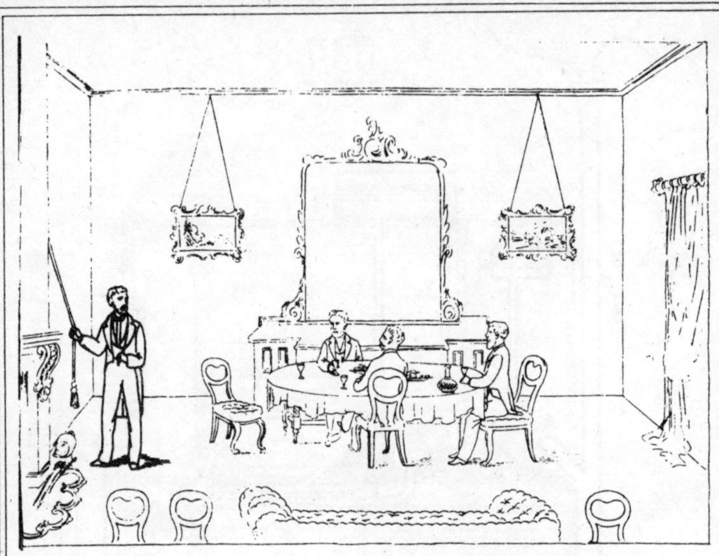

More wine wanted. Where *is* the butler?

'A lower deep,
Still threatening to devour me opens wide.'
Milton

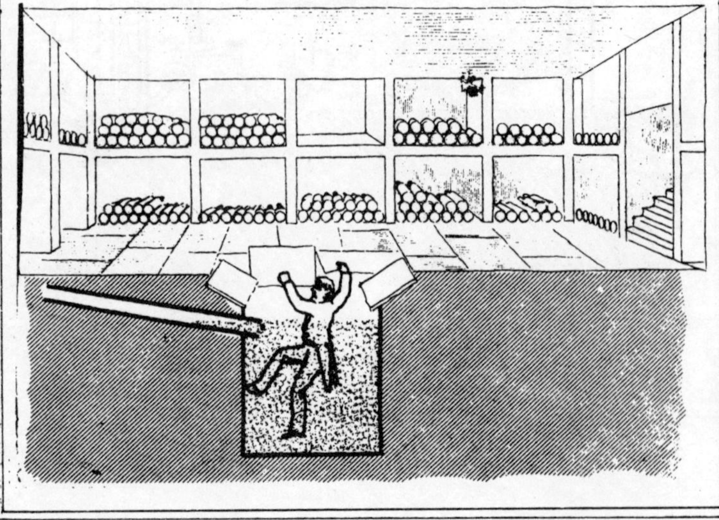

WHERE IS THE BUTLER?

A gentleman came to reside in an old family mansion. Having friends to dinner one evening, and requiring more wine, he rang the bell. No butler came. He rang a second and third time with the same result. Waxing wroth, he went in search, but could get no tidings of him. On further search the butler was discovered in an old cesspool in the wine cellar, the floor of which had broken in. The poor butler, after much difficulty, was extricated, only just in time for his life to be saved after much suffering and a month of medical attendance. It appears that the existence of this cesspool was unknown, and that so long as the sewage of the house went 'somewhere,' no enquiries were made to ascertain where.

A similar fact was told to me by a lady, as having occurred in a large house at Brighton. A cask of beer was being rolled along the cellar, when the floor gave way over an unsuspected cesspool.

Moral. Test all the floors of your cellars by 'sounding.'—*Ibid.*

Had I the compelling power there should not be a milliner, corset-maker, or *marchande de mode* in all the land entitled to practise her profession without having previously entered to three courses of lectures at the least on the science of physiology; in order that being made acquainted with the murderous work they are about to perpetrate they should not afterwards assign in extenuation innocence of intent or ignorance of the effects of those barbarities of civilization which are displayed in fashioning female costume.

I cannot but advert to that instrument of torture and premature destruction *stays*, and I know it is necessary to approach the subject as gingerly as may be. The flexibility of the ribs admits of their contraction by artificial means; and when pressure is applied externally the cavern of the chest is of course proportionally lessened in capacity. The chest, as before stated, is the habitation of the lungs, and from the peculiarity in action of that organ an ever-continuous expansion and contraction are necessary to the performance of their functions.

Now, with all possible respect to those non-natural dames whose vocation is in the concoction of corsettes, I would ask them whether any contrivance could be more capitally devised to obstruct the functions of the lungs (and, by obstructing them, destroy life) than a pair of corsettes—if I am right in assuming they go in pairs. I do not go to impute to these *artistes* a wilful intention either to destroy life or to impair health; neither is it my business to enquire into the motives by which they are actuated. 'Support,' I believe, is the assigned reason; but the philosophy of that support which of necessity *distorts* is not of easy comprehension. It is remarkable with what pertinacity art desires to reverse nature; if the configuration of the chest be regarded, it will be seen that the lowermost portion of it is far and away the largest in diameter:—on the other hand, if you will notice the first young lady of fashion you may meet in Regent Street, you shall find that *art*—perverse, envious, invidious, revolutionising art—has turned nature altogether topsy-turvy, the configuration being totally reversed, as is illustrated by the annexed diagrams.

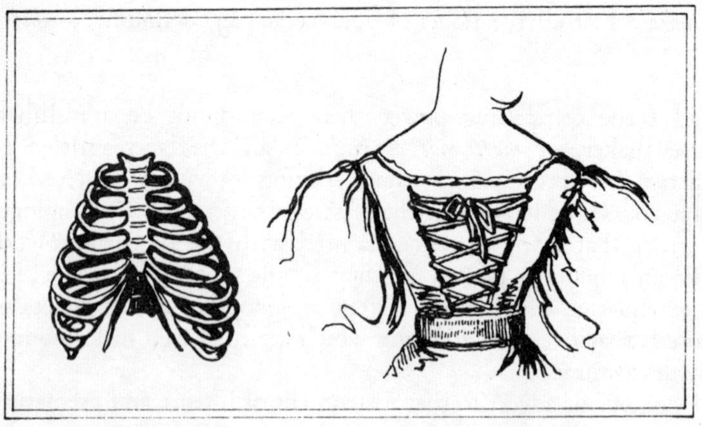

'Look here upon this picture! And on this!'

It is clear as daylight that something must give way under this new *regime*: either the lungs, which occupy so great an extent of the chest, must waste away to impart a *waist* as *waists* go in these days, or the heart must shrink in size, or the upper ribs must be pressed outwards, or some means or another must be afforded to compensate for tight lacing.—*On Consumption, Coughs, Colds, Asthma*, 1834.

Above all things, the passage of the blood through the lungs is unable to go on properly, since the lungs are pressed together by the corset, but the desire to make oneself, by means of the corset, more slender than nature has willed it, has not only caused many diseases, but has frequently been the direct cause of death.

Every day, during the ball season, one hears that here and there a lady has suddenly broken down in the middle of a dance, and, according to the medical opinion, has died from paralysis of the heart consequent upon tight-lacing, and not all of such sad cases by a long way get into the papers, for some of the sufferers escape with their life, and shame will not, as a rule, allow them to let it be known how they have been punished for their vanity. Vanity, yes, that is it, that is the root of the evil. The mothers, who have themselves not been properly brought up, also train their daughters to cripple and deform themselves.

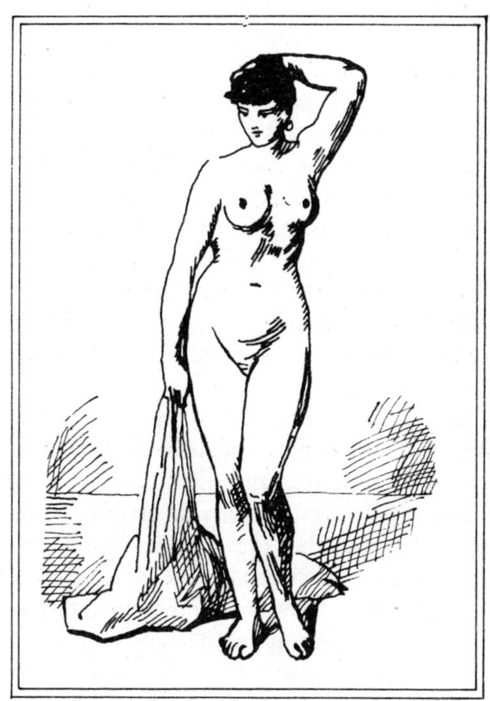

The natural bodily form of woman.

Can it be seriously believed that the laws of nature allow themselves for any length of time to be defied with impunity? Whoever has had the opportunity of seeing a tightly-laced lady undressed in the evening, will have remarked that the moment the stays fall off, a deep, happy sigh of relief is wrung from the pained breast, and not seldom there is added, internally, 'Thank heaven!'—*New Curative Treatment of Disease*, 1901.

Besides the prevention of disease, one of the great aims of the science of public health is, or most undoubtedly ought to be, the improvement of the race. We have only to look at the children—pale, wretched, pinched, crooked-limbed, and fighting with disease—who swarm in the London streets, and compare them with the sturdy, rosy-cheeked boys and girls that one encounters in well-cared-for country districts, to be sure that the town-bred children of the poor whose resources are not sufficient to counteract the adverse surroundings which encompass them, must be vastly inferior as citizens—physically as well as morally— to the children who enjoy from their birth all the advantages of fresh air, free exercise, and healthy parentage.

The theory of 'natural selection,' broached a few years since, ought certainly to have a great influence upon the science of public health, and upon the enactments which may be necessary for the forwarding of that science. According to the theories of natural selection, the weak members of a family are sure to be worsted in the battle of life, and the strong will alone survive the struggle and bear off the rewards of victory. In this way the gradual improvement of the race is insured by the eradication of the weeds and the giving of more room for the healthy plants to flourish in.

Now, the science of public health must have the effect, and doubtless has had the effect, of lessening the enemies with which man has to contend, and thus there can be no doubt that many more sickly weeds survive to manhood than formerly; and, therefore, against the great good which public health enactments doubtlessly effect for us, must be placed the counter-balancing reflection that excessive protection interferes with that process which bears good fruit in the long run—I mean 'natural selection.'

'To Plato,' says Lord Macaulay, 'the science of medicine appeared to be of very disputable advantage. He did not, indeed, object to quick cures for acute disorders, or for injuries produced by accidents; but the art which resists the slow sap of a chronic disease, which repairs frames enervated by lust, swollen by gluttony, or inflamed by wine—which encourages sensuality by mitigating the natural punishment of the sensualist, and prolongs existence when the intellect has ceased to retain its entire energy—had no share of his esteem.' 'The exercise of the art of medicine ought', he said, 'to be tolerated so far as that art may serve to cure the occasional distempers of men whose constitutions are good. As to those who have bad constitutions, let them die; and the sooner the better.'

We cherish our weeds. The patient with mental disease is allowed to go abroad as soon as the solicitous care of the physician has restored to him his reason; the hardest and most inveterate scoundrels in our prisons are often set at liberty with a ticket of leave; prostitutes are still permitted, except in a few favoured localities, to ply their calling and disseminate disease without restraint; and it is hardly too much to say that the hangman's office has become a sinecure. We adopt the same tactics with mental and moral diseases as we do with physical maladies, and in our treatment of them we are actuated by the feeling that prevention is better than cure. And so indeed it is; and no one will deny that, for all concerned—the healthy as well as the sick and erring—the less harsh we are in the treatment of our unfortunate brethren, the better. It is certainly more rational, more humane, and more in accordance with Christian doctrine, to prevent than to be ready to adopt capital measures for eradication.

The only objection which can be raised against our humane course of action arises from the knowledge that much disease, both of mind and body, is hereditary; and when we reflect that the consumptive when he leaves the hospital, the madman when he quits the asylum, and the habitual criminal when he gets his discharge or ticket of leave, are all capable of transmitting their several taints to generations yet unborn, we can hardly repress the doubt which arises in our minds as to whether Plato was not in the right after all.—*The Family Physician*, 1883.

10

Some Methods of Treatment of Use to the Diligent Physician

Any one who has seen Leeches used knows how difficult it is sometimes to get them to bite readily; and the old nurses can tell you how they seem to be possessed with a spirit of contradiction. They will either refuse to bite at all, or will fasten anywhere but on the desired spot. All sorts of instructions are given in books, but most of them are useless. A leech partakes to some extent of the nature of a fish, that is, it lives in water; and therefore, instead of holding them in a warm hand or a dry towel, act in this way:

First wash the place perfectly clean, then put your leeches into a wineglass, and fill it with water; put a piece of paper over it, turn the glass upside down on to the place where you want them to fix, and draw the paper away; you will find now that the leeches being in their native element, are cool and comfortable, and will settle instantly, thereby saving a great amount of vexation and loss of time. As soon as they have taken hold, place a towel round the glass to soak up the water, and remove it. In this way you get them exactly where you wish, either all on one spot or distributed over a larger space, by putting on only one or two at a time. If you require one on a very particular spot, for instance, close to the eye, and have not a proper leech-glass, put it tail first into a small narrow phial filled with water. Where they have to be used inside the mouth, nostrils, etc., it is better to pass a needleful of thread through the tail to hold by; it will not prevent them biting; and if one should be swallowed, drink a little salt and water. Leeches are always expensive, but with a little care they need not be destroyed. When they come off do not dip them into salt; put them into a large jar of water, with an inch or two of turf or garden soil; change the water every day for the first week, then once a week will be sufficient; in this they will clear themselves and recover. Any

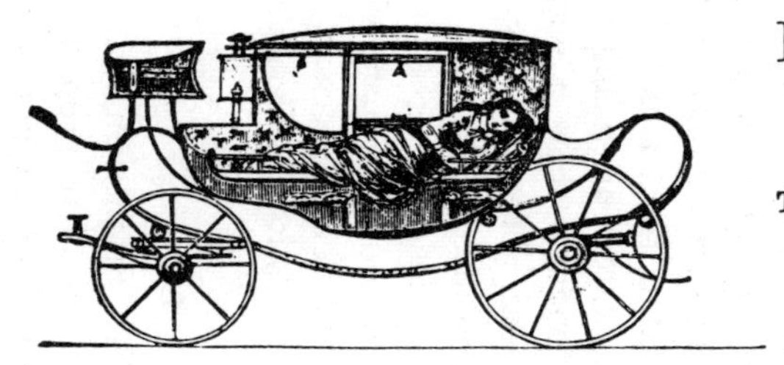

IMPROVED INVALID COT CARRIAGES.

THE GREATEST LUXURY AND COMFORT EVER INTRODUCED FOR REMOVING INVALIDS, BEING FITTED UP WITH THE

PATENT NOISELESS WHEELS.

These Carriages may be engaged, on moderate terms, for any journey, on application to

H. & J. READING,

COACHBUILDERS, 14, RIDING HOUSE-STREET, CAVENDISH-SQUARE.

N.B. A good assortment of New and Second-hand Carriages for Sale or Hire.

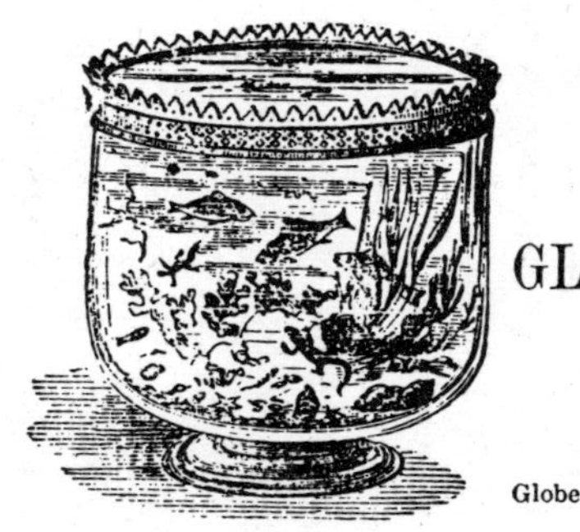

AQUARIA FOR FISH OR LEECHES,

In a Variety of Shapes and Sizes,

AT

CLAUDET AND HOUGHTON'S

GLASS-SHADE AND WINDOW-GLASS WAREHOUSE,

89, HIGH HOLBORN, LONDON.

LISTS OF PRICES SENT FREE ON APPLICATION.

N.B.—The Aquaria may be advantageously applied to the keeping of Leeches.

Globe Aquarium, 13 in. diameter, suitable for about 100 Leeches, 13s.; or fitted with suitable Plants and Snails, 17s. 6d. Ditto, 16 inches, for 200 Leeches, 16s. 6d.; or with Plants and Snails, £1 2s. 6d.

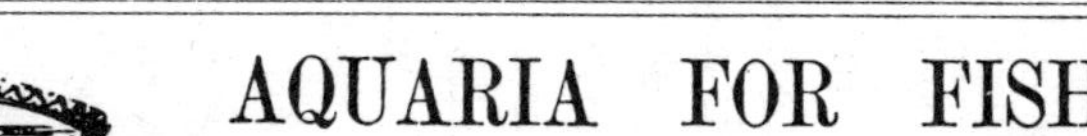
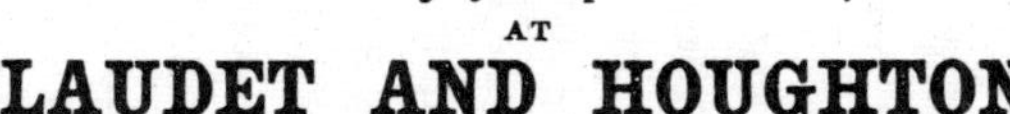

dead ones must be removed, or they will spoil the water and destroy the others.—*Till the Doctor Comes*, 1870.

Leeches are very delicate animals, and bear handling very badly; the nurse must therefore be careful not to subject them to any rough usage, or they will possibly die or prove of no use. It is often difficult to get a leech to bite, and the most common cause of such a refusal is that the skin of the patient has not been properly cleansed before applying the leech. It is recommended by some that if the leech still refuses to bite the skin should be moistened with a little milk, cream, or sugar and water. Miss Veitch says that she once succeeded in persuading an obstinate leech to bite by putting it for a few moments into a basin with a little beer. When applying leeches they should be held delicately by the tail, but care must be taken not in any way to bruise them. Special tubes of glass called leech-glasses are sold, into which the leeches are to be placed when applying them, but care is required, lest the wrong end of the leech be put into the bottom of the tube. The leech is very similar at both ends, but the mouth is known by its presenting an appearance of three rays. A leech is said when in health to be able to extract about a fluid drachm of blood. If it be thought desirable to encourage the flow of blood, this may be done by applying poultices or hot fomentations to the part, and bleeding may be kept up for some time from a leech-bite in this way. It occasionally happens, on the other hand, that the bleeding from a leech-bite is too profuse, and this may even go to the extent of endangering life, for there is nothing in which individuals show a wider difference than in the disposition to bleed. The best way to check excessive bleeding is to apply pressure to the part by means of a compress made of lint. If this does not serve, it is recommended to apply a matico leaf, or to touch the part with caustic. Cases are recorded in which it has been necessary to bring the edges of the bite together with a stitch.—*The Family Physician*, 1883.

Animal Magnetism, Curative Magnetism. By magnetism, in the inner sense of the word, is meant the peculiar property of certain bodies of attracting iron. Those which already possess this power in their natural state, as the magnet stone, are called natural magnets. Those which have acquired it through artificial treatment are termed artificial magnets. In early times, natural magnets, especially the magnetic stone, were used as curative agents, very frequently in the treatment of cramp.

The magnet is placed on the affected part of the body for from fifteen to thirty minutes, the part affected being at the same time turned towards the north, while the south pole of the magnet is placed in such a manner that its north pole is directed towards the north. In other cases on the contrary, the magnetic stone was constantly carried about on the body. It was bound to the chest in large flat pieces, or to the abdomen, limbs, &c., or worn in the form of necklets, bracelets, etc., these being inlaid with minute portions of the stone.

This curative treatment was founded on mineral magnetism. Analogous to the laws by which iron is attracted to the magnet, the attractive power which draws all bodies towards each other was already, in primitive times, connected with magnetism. For maintaining a harmonious balance between the organic and inorganic worlds, some common power was supposed to exist, as connecting medium between body and soul, light and matter, motion and rest. This magnetic influence worked between organic bodies, men, animals, and plants, and especially, in perfection, between man and man. The attraction existing between living bodies was termed animal magnetism.

Paracelsus, who reintroduced the science, was the first to connect magnetism with physics, and he held that all mutual attractions were magnetic. He speaks of magnetism, magnetic power, and magnetic mysteries. 'Man,' he says, 'possesses a hidden power, which, in one way, may be compared to a magnet, for by it he draws from surrounding chaos the possibility of infection through the air. Man possesses a magnetism without which he cannot exist, and the said magnetism exists on account of the man, not vice versa; and further, it is of stellar descent.' So far Theophrastus Paracelsus. Everyone thus possesses the power of influencing, either voluntarily or involuntarily, those with whom he comes in contact.—*New Curative Treatment of Disease*, 1901.

Local bloodletting is chiefly applicable as an auxiliary to general bloodletting, and in local diseases in which general bloodletting is not required. In cases of inflammation within the head, chest, or abdomen, after the due abstraction of blood generally, the local abstraction of blood is very often employed most opportunely. The second remedy secures the benefit, which the first had conferred. In regard to the application of a large number of leeches in such cases, a few words of caution are, however, necessary. The loss of the blood so withdrawn is not always well borne when the lancet has been used efficiently just before; and if applied late at night, the flow of blood is apt to continue unheeded, until an undue quantity of blood has been poured out. Both these events have occurred, and led to unavailing regret.

Cupping is, generally speaking, a more efficient remedy than leeching. It is most appropriately applied to the nape of the neck, behind the ears, to the temples, to the various parts of the chest, over the region of the liver, the kidney, &c. To the softer parts of the abdomen, leeches must be applied.

Both these remedies are peculiarly efficacious in cases in which the powers of the whole system have been duly subdued by general bloodletting, without the removal of the symptoms of the local disease. Only the quantity so withdrawn after the general bloodletting must not be too great.

In some chronic local affections, in which general bloodletting would be inadmissible, the local abstraction of blood by leeches or cupping becomes our chief remedy. Such cases are chronic inflammation within the head, thorax, or abdomen; especially when this is fixed chiefly to one part or organ. Inflammatory pain long confined to one part of the head or chest, chronic inflammation of the liver, kidney, uterus, &c. are cases in which local bloodletting is the appropriate remedy.

It should not be omitted, perhaps, that the application of leeches near the anus has been much recommended in France, in order to effect what is supposed to be effected by hemorrhoidal discharges, viz. to unload the vena portæ, and to relieve the head or the liver. This mode of local bloodletting is also very beneficial in diarrhœa and dysentery. Leeches have also been applied by means of an appropriate metallic tube to the vagina or to the os uteri, in cases of inflammation of those parts.

These appear to be appropriate cases for the use of local bloodletting by cupping and leeches. Scarification is a mode of taking blood in a few cases of local disease, as in inflammation of the eye, of the tonsils, and in inflamed hemorrhoids.—*The Cyclopaedia of Practical Medicine*, 1833.

Several vegetable juices produce an eruption of small blisters; as that of some kinds of ranunculus, clematis, &c. But the Spanish blistering-fly, the *cantharis*, or *meloë vesicatoria*, is the remedy which best answers as a vesicant, and is the one almost solely employed. The active property, according to the researches of Robiquet, appears to reside in a peculiar principle soluble in æther and in oil, to which is applied the name of *cantharidin*. The form, therefore, in which it is most successfully applied is in a compound of the powdered flies with hog's lard, or some such oleaginous substance, and a due proportion of wax or resin to give it the consistence of soft plaster. This spread on leather, or any other convenient substance, and applied to the skin, soon produces a sense of heat and pricking in the part, attended, if the application is large, with some excitement of the circulation and quickness of the pulse. If it be removed in two or three hours, its effect is merely rubefacient, and no blistering is produced; but if it be allowed to remain for a space varying in different individuals from five to ten hours, the skin will be found raised in large blisters filled with a yellowish serum, which continue to rise after the blister has been removed. In some cases they do not appear until after it has been dressed; and it is, therefore, unnecessary to keep the plaster on until they are formed, or till, as it is commonly expressed, the blister rises. When the blisters are fully risen, they are snipped with a pair of scissors, which allows the serum to escape; and if it be intended that the part should heal, it is dressed with simple ointment spread on a linen rag. The serosity continues to escape, and sometimes to raise fresh blisters, for some hours after; these must be treated as before, and the dressing renewed twice in twenty-four hours. When, from peculiar idiosyncrasy, blisters produce great irritation, local or general, the addition of a little powdered opium or acetate of morphia to the plaster may give relief. An excess of inflammation, which occasionally ensues after the rising of a blister, sometimes with erysipelatous or eczematous appearances around it, is best relieved by poultices, which are proper applications whenever it is desirable to moderate the irritation. When the blistered part shows a disposition to gangrene, which is not unfrequently the case with children, it must be treated on general principles, as by stimulating or other applications, solutions of chloride of lime or soda, and bark exhibited internally. To avoid this consequence in children, it is advisable never to allow the blister to remain on more than six hours; and a poultice should be substituted if the inflammation be at all high.—*Ibid.*

Baunschedit constructed an instrument for the production of a kind of artificial gnat-sting in the skin, and invented an oil which was similar in its composition to the fluid given forth by the gnats when they sting. To this instrument he gave the name of 'Re-vitalizer'. This consists of a small cylindrical hollow shaft of ebony, about six inches in length. At the upper end it broadens out into a club, out of which projects a circular surface about half-an-inch in diameter, containing thirty-three steel needles, which project about one centimetre in length. On the other side of the club is a spiral spring, which lies in the narrow hollow space of the shaft, and which projects out of the lower side of this shaft, having a handle attached to it. When the instrument is not in use, the needles do not project beyond the circumference of the club-like end of the tube. When the apparatus is to be used, this upper part of the club end is pressed close on to the skin, the spiral spring is caught hold of by the projecting handle, drawn back, and then suddenly released. This causes the thirty-three needles to strike suddenly into the skin, more or less deeply, according to the force employed. There is, however, no appreciable feeling of pain caused by the punctures, because the needles immediately spring back after their impact, moreover, there is no bleeding whatever from the punctures.

The composition of the oil (Oleum Baunscheidtii) its inventor kept secret, and the recipe for this oil was, after his death, only communicated to his family on the condition of their keeping the secret, and retaining it as hereditary property in the family.

By the application of this instrument on the human skin, there at first arises a local effect, viz., a relaxation of the epidermis (our outer skin which protects the real skin); a slight wounding of the dermal tissue, or the true skin itself; and an increased circulation of blood through the skin . . . .—*New Curative Treatment of Disease*, 1901.

As a remedial agent, electricity may be applied in five different ways. The first method, which is, we believe, at present employed is to *excite* the patient by placing him upon an insulating stool, and putting him in connexion with the prime conductor of a machine in action. This is what is called the electric *bath*. It was strongly recommended by Priestly, apparently under the impression adopted from the Abbé Nollet, that the animal functions are, under such circumstances, discharged with increased vigour, particularly the circulation of the blood and the cutaneous secretion. Such effects are sometimes observed, but by no means invariably. The bath was employed by Lit and De Haen, two early writers upon medical electricity, for the treatment of hysteria.

The next and simplest method of applying electricity to the cure of disease is to present the member, or part affected, to the prime conductor of the machine, and thus cause it to receive a succession of sparks; or, what is more convenient, to place the patient on a chair, and convey to him the sparks by means of a director connected with the conductor by a chain. The patient may manage the director while the operator works the machine.

The third mode consists in placing the patient upon an insulating stool, putting him in connexion, through means of a chain or metallic rod, with the prime conductor, and drawing sparks from the seat of disease or pain by simply presenting to such part the knuckle, or, should the operator dislike receiving the spark himself, an uninsulated director. This method of operating has the advantage over the preceding that it conjoins the electrical bath with the influence of the spark. It is, therefore, that usually adopted by those experienced in the medicinal administration of electricity. The force of the spark is proportionate to its length, so that, by properly diminishing this, its strength may be reduced to any required standard.

A favourite mode with some practitioners of applying sparks is to *give* or *draw* them across flannel. For this purpose, a director, terminated by a large ball, which is to be covered with a fold of flannel, is approached in the usual way to the organ to be electrified. Instead of a single strong spark, a series of weak ones will thus be produced, which, emanating at the same instant from several of the woollen fibres, extend over a considerable surface and produce in it a peculiar pricking sensation. The ball of the director may be naked, the flannel being laid on the part of the body which is to be submitted to the influence of the sparks. This method is supposed to be particularly suited to the treatment of rheumatism and paralysis, especially in patients who cannot endure the stronger forms of electricity.

The next form of medical electricity to be noticed is the *aura*, or jet of air, which proceeds from an electrified point. This is the modification of the electric influence to which ulcers, excoriated surfaces, and delicate organs, such as the eye and testicle, are usually subjected. The common method of employing the aura is to present a pointed director, connected by a chain, with the conductor of the machine, and held by a glass handle, to the part affected. The particles of air in contact with the point are highly electrified, and, of course, immediately repelled. The same occurs to those which take their place, and so on in succession, producing a current of highly excited air, which, as has been just described, is directed upon the organ which is the subject of electrical treatment. The aura may also be applied by placing the patient upon an insulating stool, and directing an uninsulated pointed director to the seat of disease. It is, however, seldom resorted to, as its efficacy is more than questionable.—*The Cyclopaedia of Practical Medicine*, 1833.

When on the high road to recovery, the sufferer from liver disorder will often derive benefit from the use of the nitro-muriatic acid bath. This is prepared by adding two ounces of strong hydrochloric and one ounce of strong nitric acid to two gallons of water, at a temperature of 96 or 98 degrees. Both feet are to be placed in the bath, while the legs and thighs, the region over the liver, and both arms, are sponged alternately, or the abdomen may be swathed in flannel soaked in the water. The process is to be continued for half an hour night and morning. It is absolutely necessary that a wooden tub should be used, as the acid very soon destroys any ordinary metal bath. The sponges and towels should be placed in cold water after use, or they too will soon be destroyed.—*The Family Physician*, 1883.

The peat bog is carried to the neighbourhood of the baths, and there allowed to dry to some extent. It is then sifted and separated from the woody fibres and coarser materials, when it is mixed with the mineral water of the Louisenquelle into the consistence of a very soft poultice. In this state it is heated by steam to a temperature varying from 80° to 100° of Fahrenheit, when it is ready for the bather, being worked up by means of wooden instruments and the hands into a complete black amalgam. I took the mud-bath here, at Marienbad, and Carlsbad, and do not regret the experiments. I confess that, at first, I felt some repugnance, not fear, in plunging into the black peat poultice; but when up to the chin (temperature 97°) I felt more comfortable than I had ever done, even in the baths of Schlangenbad, Wildbad, or Pfeffers. The material is so dense, that you are some time in sinking to the bottom of the bath—and I could not help fancying myself in Mahomet's tomb, suspended between Heaven and Earth, but possessing consciousness, which I fear the prophet did not enjoy.

There was one drawback on the mud-bath, or peat-poultice. We cannot roll about, like a porpoise or whale, as in the water-bath, without considerable effort, so dense is the medium in which we lie; but I found that I could use friction to all parts of the body, with great ease, in consequence of the unctuous and lubricating quality of the bath. After twenty minutes' immersion, I felt an excitement of the surface, quite different from that of the common mineral warm baths—even of those of Wisbaden, Kissengen, or Schwalbach—attended, as I fancied, by elevation of spirits.

Here and at other spas where mud-baths are employed, I met with several veteran warriors, whose aching wounds reminded them too often of battlefields and bloody campaigns. They almost all agreed in attributing more efficacy to these than to the common baths—and I think, from what I have seen, heard, and felt, that there is much truth in these statements. The Schlamm-bads have one advantage over the others, which is more prized on the Continent than in England—the facilities which they afford the bathers, both male and female, of receiving morning visits from their friends while in the mud, and that without any violation of delicacy, propriety, or decorum; for there, persons are more completely veiled than in any dress, even of the most dense and sable furs of Russia. An English lady of rank, at Teplitz, was visited by her physician and friends while immersed to the chin in peat-bog. They read to her, and conversed with her till the signal was given for exchanging the black varnish for the limpid and purifying wave, when they retired.—*Pilgrimages to the Spas*, 1841.

Hot air baths and vapour baths can with a little ingenuity be administered in a private house. The hot air bath is managed by placing in the patient's bed under the clothes a great Davy's lamp, so constructed that the bed-clothes are kept well off the lamp. This arrangement is perfectly safe, and so successful that in a very short time the maximum temperature that the patient

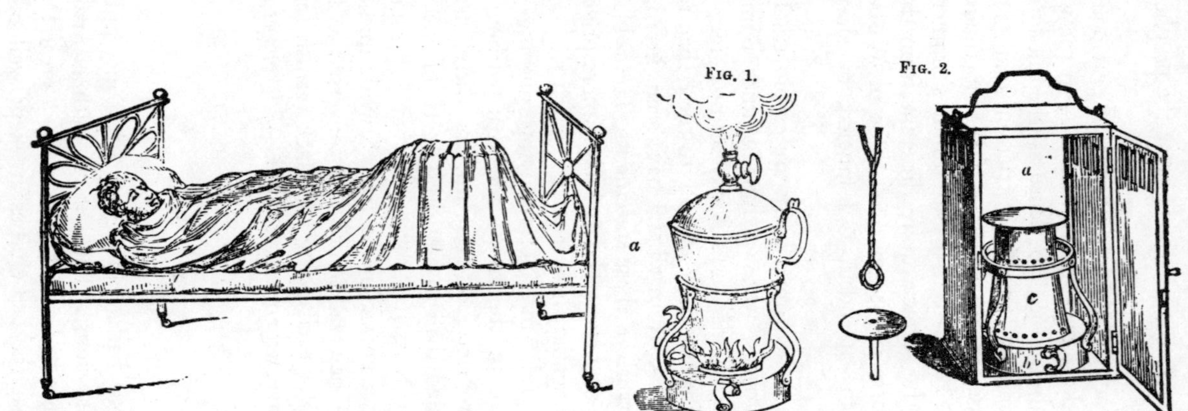

NOEDL'S PATENT VAPOUR-BATH.—A thoroughly effective, portable VAPOUR-BATH, at a moderate cost, approved and recommended by several eminent Medical Gentlemen. The apparatus can be placed with perfect safety beneath the bed-clothes, close to the patient. (See Woodcut.) It maintains a uniform heat, and can be applied without trouble, being very simple in its construction.

Description of the Apparatus as applied for Steam or Medicated Vapour.—Fig. 1, the Vapour Generator; *a*, the Boiler; *b*, the Spirit Lamp. The Apparatus for Hot Air, Fig. 2; *b*, the Spirit Lamp, placed in Perforated Safe, *a*: *c*, a Cylinder for confining the Spirit Flame in a small compass.

Manufactured and Sold Wholesale by **BENHAMS & FROUD, 40, 41, & 42, Chandos-street, Charing-cross**; to be obtained Retail of all respectable Ironmongers. — Illustrated Prospectuses, with full details, sent post-free. — A liberal Discount to the Profession.

can bear is reached. Whenever an arrangement of this kind is employed, the patient should lie between the blankets, in order that the very copious perspiration which will assuredly result may be thoroughly absorbed, and the patient run no chance of a chill. A vapour bath requires only a very simple contrivance: an ordinary washing-tub should be fitted with a false bottom, and over it should be hung a circular curtain made of flannel, and having a metal top like the curtain of a shower bath. An ordinary large kettle should then be fitted with a long tin pipe conducting the steam from the spout of the kettle to the tub below the false bottom, which is perforated to let the steam pass upwards.—*The Family Physician*, 1883.

I would likewise observe, that the real Quantity of animal Fluid carried off by Perspiration, can never be known by Ponderation; for it is plain that the outward Air enters the pores of the Body and is sometimes imbib'd or absorb'd by the Animal, the Quantity of perspirable Matter is only the Difference of the Excess of that beyond the Quantity of Air that is imbib'd.—*The Effect of Air on Human Bodies*, 1733.

In recommending to his followers the use of water, Mr Wesley proceeds to state, *that cold bathing cures young children of the following complaints:*—

Convulsions, coughs, gravel	Pimples and scabs
Inflammations of ears, navel	Suppression of urine
and mouth	Vomiting
Rickets	Want of sleep
Cutaneous inflammations	

Water, he further adds, frequently cures every nervous and every paralytic disorder. In particular

Asthma	Lethargy
Agues of every sort	Loss of speech, taste, appetite,
Atrophy	smell
Blindness	Nephritic pains
Cancer	Palpitation of the heart
Coagulated blood of the	Pain in the back, joints
bruises	stomach

Chin cough
Consumption
Convulsions
Coughs
Complication of distempers
Convulsive pains
Deafness
Dropsy
Epilepsy
Violent fever
Gout (running)
Hectic fevers
Hysteric pains
Incubus
Inflammations
Involuntary stool or urine
Lameness
Leprosy (old)
Rheumatism
Rickets
Rupture
Suffocations
Surfeits at the beginning
Sciatica
Scorbutic pains
Swelling in the joints
Stone in the kidneys
Torpor of the limbs, even when the use of them is lost
Tetanus
Tympany
Vertigo
St Vitus's dance
Vigilia
Varicose ulcers
The Whites

Water prevents the growth of hereditary

Apoplexies
Asthmas
Blindness
Consumptions
Deafness
Gout
King's evil
Melancholy
Palsies
Rheumatism
Stone

Water drinking generally prevents

Apoplexies
Asthma
Convulsions
Gout
Hysteric fits
Madness
Palsies
Stone
Trembling

To this children should be used from their cradles.

For Asthma—Take a pint of cold water every morning, washing the head in cold water immediately after, and using the cold bath.

Rickets in Children—Dip them in cold water every morning.

To prevent apoplexy—Use the cold bath and drink only cold water.

Ague—Go into a cold bath just before the cold.

Cancer in the breast—Use the cold bath. This has cured many. This cured Mrs Bates, of Leicestershire, of a cancer in her breast, a consumption, a sciatica, and rheumatism, which she had nearly twenty years. NB Generally, where cold bathing is necessary to cure any disease, water drinking is so, to prevent a relapse.

Hysteric colic—Mrs Watts, by using the cold bath two and twenty times in a month, was entirely cured of an hysteric colic, fits, and convulsive motions, continual sweatings and vomitings, wandering pains in her limbs and head, and total loss of appetite.

To prevent the ill effects of cold—The moment a person gets into a house, with his hands and feet quite chilled, let him put them into a vessel of water, as cold as can be got, and hold them there.—*Hydropathy or the Cold Water Cure*, 1842.

SHOWER-BATHS

The shower-baths I apply are the following:
The knee shower. The legs being uncovered to the knees and the

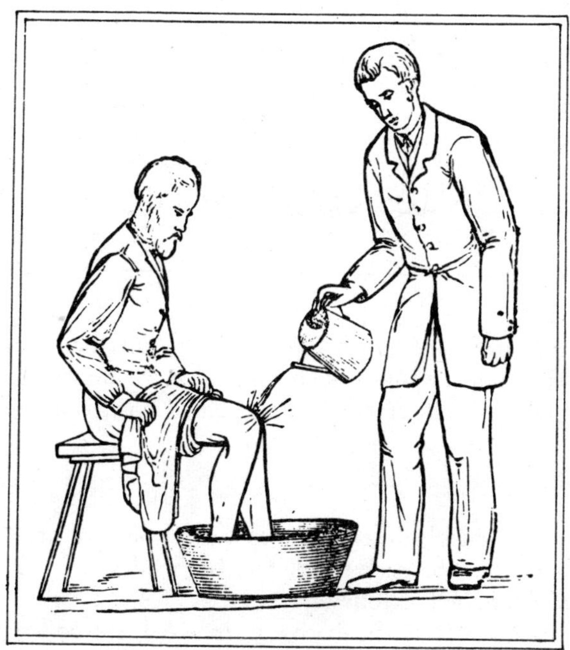

clothes kept back as far as possible to prevent their getting wet, the patient sits down on a chair, both his feet standing in a prepared vessel as if to take a foot-bath.

The shower is given by means of a small watering-can (such as is used in a green-house, which can easily be managed with one hand).

The upper shower-bath. The patient takes off all the clothing of the upper body, and, to prevent the remainder getting wet, puts a cloth round his waist. The tub into which the water is to run off, may stand on a low chair or foot-stool, instead of on the floor, in order to make the bending down easier; it serves also to spare the head, i.e. to diminish by a more upright position, the

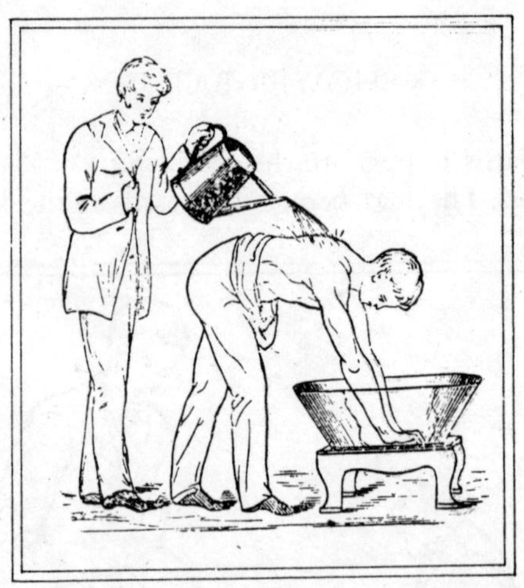

determination of blood to it. The patient leans both his hands on the bottom of the tub in such a way that the upper body takes a horizontal position, and the water poured on it can flow down into the tub.

The whole shower-bath. It extends, as the name indicates, to the whole body from the neck to the feet both sides.

It is to be applied as follows:

The patient sits in the bath, or in a wide wooden, or tin

vessel, on a small board, dressed in bathing-trousers or a bathing-shirt. The shower is given partly on the back, partly on the front, with about 4 cans of water. The first must wet the whole body. The following three or more cans are given in such a way, that the jet is directed to all parts of the body, especially to the spinal marrow and the chief sympathetics, i.e. to the nape and both sides of it, then to the pit of the stomach.

This shower may be recommended to healthy, especially corpulent persons.

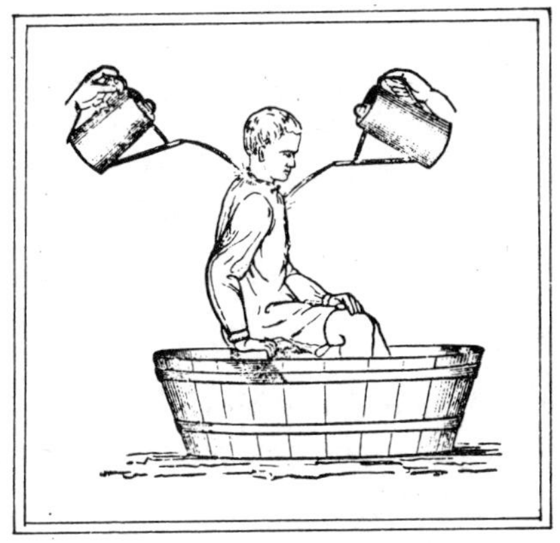

Walking in water. As simple as it may appear to walk in water reaching as far as the calf of the leg, yet even this application serves as a means of hardening; it has influence on the whole body, and strengthens the whole system; (b) it operates on the kidneys; by this many complaints, originating in the kidneys, the bladder and the bowels, are prevented, (c) it operates power-fully on the chest, facilitates breathing and carries gases out of the stomach, (d) it operates especially against heachache, con-gestion, and other sufferings of the head. This means of hardening can be employed by moving the feet in a bath of cold water, reaching over the ankles. It is more efficacious for hardening, if one goes into the water up to the shins, and most efficacious of all, if the water reaches the knees.

As to the duration, one can begin with 1 minute, then longer, up to 5 or 6 minutes. The colder the water, the better. After such a practice exercise is necessary, in winter time in a warm room, in summer in the open air, until the body is completely warm.

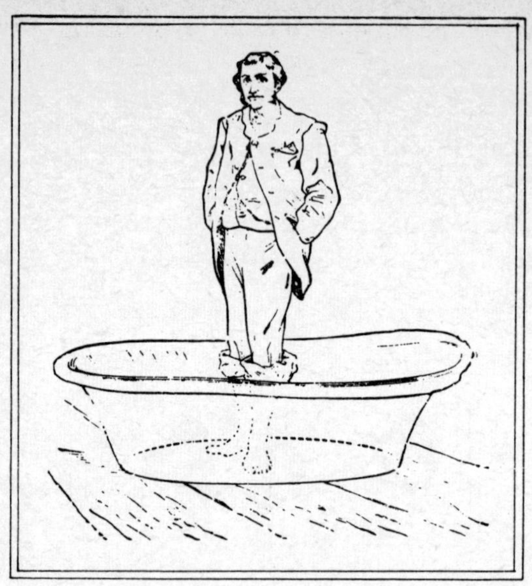

In winter, snow may be mixed with the water. With weaklings, warm water may be used in the beginning, then by and by, colder, and lastly quite cold water.

The head-bath. The head-bath belongs to the most important part-baths. It is best taken, cold or warm, in the following way:

A vessel with water is put on a chair, and the upper part of the head, the proper soil of the hair, is put into the cold water

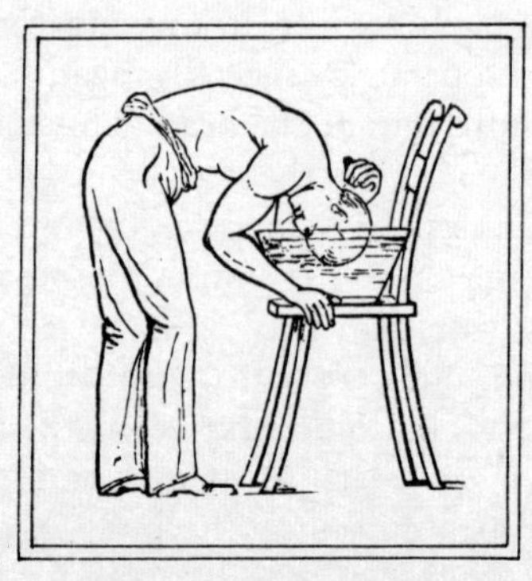

for about one minute, but if it is taken in warm water, for 5 to 7 minutes. Where the water does not reach the hair, it may be supplied with the hand, in order to wet all the hair.

After the bath, the hair must be very carefully dried. And this should never be omitted whether the hair has become wet through the shower or through the vapour. Great care and exactness should be observed; otherwise serious complaints of the head, such as rheumatism, would likely ensue. After the drying one remains in the room, or puts on a cap or bonnet large enough to cover the whole of the wet hair, until the skin of the head and the hair are perfectly dry.—*My Water Cure*, 1892.

A. B., a woman of about sixty years of age, who lived with her brother, in the county of Down, retired one evening to bed with her daughter, both being, as was their constant habit, in a state of intoxication. A little before day some members of the family were awakened by an extremely offensive smoke which pervaded their apartment, and on going into the chamber where the old woman and her daughter slept, they found the smoke to proceed from the body of the former, which appeared to be burning with an internal fire. It was as black as coal, and the smoke issued from every part of it. The combustion having been arrested, which was effected with difficulty, although there was no flame, life was found completely extinct. While the body was being removed into the coffin, which was done as soon as possible, it was dropping in pieces. Her daughter, who slept in the same bed, sustained no injury; nor did the combustion extend to the bed or bed-clothes, which exhibited no other traces of fire than the stains produced by the smoke. According to the testimony of one of the relations, who is represented as a woman of the strictest veracity, there was no fire whatever in the room. The subject of this case had been grossly intemperate for several days before her decease, having drunk at this period much more ardent spirit than usual.

From the case just related, and several others which might be quoted from the writings of Vic D'Azyr, Lecat, Lair, Kopp, Dupuytren, and Marc, it would appear fully proved that the human body is capable of being reduced to such a state as to undergo spontaneously, or upon the contact of flame, rapid changes analogous to those which may be effected by the agency of fire. A careful examination, also, of the histories of the several instances upon record, has enabled us to collect, at least with some probability, the circumstances which precede, accompany, and characterize this malady; for such it obviously must be considered. These we shall now enumerate, as they will serve as a guide to our inquiries respecting the immediate or proximate cause of the phenomenon.

1. Spontaneous combustion would appear to be a calamity almost peculiar to the old and feeble; for it has seldom occurred to persons of a robust constitution, or under sixty years of age.

2. Women seem particularly prone to it. Thus, of the seventeen cases collected by Kopp, sixteen occurred to females, while the subjects of the eight cases mentioned by Lair are all of the same sex.

3. Individuals who have thus suffered have, generally speaking, been remarkable for the inactivity of their habits, for corpulency, or the opposite state, great emaciation, and for their inordinate use of spirituous liquors.

Of the circumstances which distinguish spontaneous from ordinary combustion, the following seem most deserving of notice.

1. The combustion spreads with extraordinary rapidity; the decomposition of the entire body being usually effected in an extremely short period of time.

2. The flame is of a lambent and flickering nature, of a blue colour, very difficult to extinguish by water, and not readily communicable to inflammable bodies placed in its vicinity.

3. A strong empyreumatic odour is usually exhaled, and there is found upon adjacent objects a fetid and moist fuliginous deposit, of a greasy nature.

4. The trunk is generally entirely consumed, but portions of the head and extremities are occasionally left uninjured.—*The Cyclopaedia of Practical Medicine*, 1833.

11

To Prepare Some Useful Recipes for the Treatment of Disease

Do not confound low price and cheapness together. They are very different, especially in important things like medicines. If you insist upon paying a very low price for an article, you drive the seller to give you either what is kept till it has become useless, or what is adulterated. I will tell you an anecdote. I was writing a prescription in a chemist's shop, when a child came in with a small packet in her hand, and said, 'Please, mister, mother says you've cheated her shameful with this magnesia, she can get twice as much for a penny at the other druggist's.' So he gave her double the quantity, and said to her, 'Be sure to tell your mother that the other was stronger, and so I gave her less of it.'

When she was gone, he said to me, 'Now here is a difficult case. You doctors blame us for not selling pure drugs. I gave

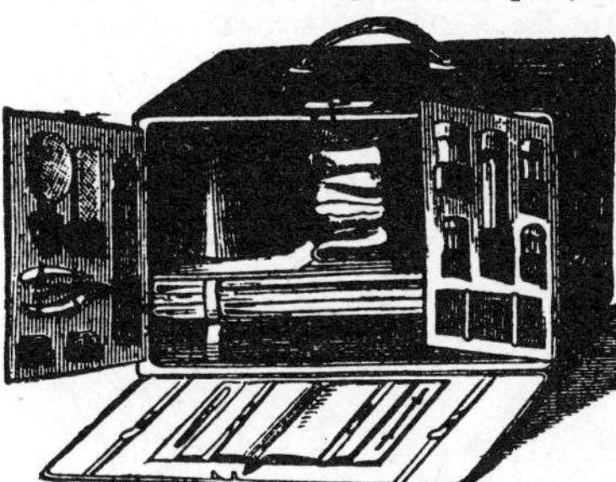

NEW TRAVELLING BAG PORTMANTEAU, the "Duke of Edinburgh," is the most marvellously compact-fitted bag ever yet invented. By means of shelves, which are supplied with the bag, it can be packed like a Cabinet, and when open (see Engraving) every article is exposed to view. The fittings occupy the folding wings, and comprise four glass bottles for oil, brushes, soap and scent, Hair Brush, Hat Brush, Razors, Scissors, Strop, Nail-cleaner, Box of Matches, Writing-pad, Penholder, Pencil-case, Paper-knife, Writing Paper, &c. Price complete, £5 5s.; larger sizes, £6 6s., £7 7s. Without flap, wings, and fittings, £2 2s., £2 10s., £3 3s. Surgical instruments can be packed on the folding wings in extra elastic bands fitted on for that purpose, rendering the portmanteau bag invaluable for doctors whilst travelling. For illustration of novelties in Portmanteaus, Travelling Bags, &c., see "Our Magazine of Useful Novelties, Presents, and Inventions," 6 stamps.

her as much pure magnesia for her penny as I could afford; but she must have more bulk, so I am compelled to mix a quantity of chalk with it; and now she goes away boasting that she has taught the druggist a lesson not to try to cheat people.'

The consequence of this system is, that if the patient takes only the dose the doctor ordered, the medicine has not the proper effect, and in case of serious illness the time for doing good may be gone by, and a life be lost in consequence.

You must be very careful about the size of the dose, especially if you give it without a doctor's orders. Medicine given at random is as likely to kill as to cure.—*Till the Doctor Comes*, 1870.

In administering powders it should be borne in mind that the act of swallowing is mainly an involuntary one, and that if the materials to be swallowed be placed far enough back in the throat they must continue their journey to the stomach whether the patient desire it or not. Powders therefore should be placed quite upon the back of the tongue, beyond what are technically known as the pillars of the fauces—*i.e.*, the two bands which, on looking into the mouth, may be seen stretching from the uvula to the tongue on either side. That horrible instrument of torture which formerly was regarded as an household requisite, but which happily is becoming daily more and more rare—we mean the *physic spoon*—was constructed on purpose for the administration of powders. It consisted of a spoon with a lid and a hollow handle, and it was only necessary to introduce the spoon into the mouth—into which it exactly fitted—when, on blowing down the handle of the spoon, the contents of it were left safely adhering to the back of the throat, whence all efforts to dislodge them proved almost absolutely futile. Powders are happily nowadays not often so bulky as formerly was the case, and it is seldom necessary to employ for their administration the formidable engine we have described.—*The Family Physician*, 1883.

A WATER AGAINST CONSUMPTIONS

Take snails fresh out of the garden, with their shells four pounds, leaves of liverwort, lungwort, ground ivy, scabious, Pauls betony, Selfheal, each six ounces, crust of bread half-a-pound, conserve

of red roses and succory flowers each twelve ounces, nutmegs
No. 6, let all be bruised together into a mash and pour upon
them of milk hot from the cow one gallon and a-half, stirring
them well together, about an hour after put to them of malaga
wine one gallon, Damask rose water two pounds, and draw off
with a sand-heat two gallons.—*West Wickham Cookery Book*, 1934.

PLAGUE WATER

Take Rue, Rosemary, Balm, Carduus, Scordium, Marigold-
Flowers, Dragons, Goats-Rue, Mint, each three Handfuls; Roots
of Master-Wort, Angelica, Butterbur, Piony, each fix Ounces;
Scorzonera, three Ounces; Proof Spirits, three Gallons: Macerate,
distil, and make it up high Proof.

ANOTHER WAY

Get the Roots of Master-Wort, Gentian, Snake Root, each two
Ounces; green Walnuts bruised, twenty-four; Venice Treacle
and Mithridate, each one Ounce; Camphire, two Drachms;
Rue, Elecampane-Root, each one Ounce; Hore-Hound, two
Ounces; Saffron, a Dram; Proof-Spirits, three Gallons; Water
sufficient: Distil, and sweeten with White Sugar one Pound and
a half for Use.

Note, That the Saffron is best added after Distillation.—*The
Lady's Companion*, 1751.

Sarsaparilla was at one time regarded almost as a 'cure-all,' and
administered in almost all chronic diseases. As a proof of its
efficacy, it was stated by its advocates that patients who com-
menced taking it often continued to do so for months or years.
This we should regard rather as a proof that it was inert, for if it
were possessed of active properties it would surely either have
killed or cured them long before. The fact is that sarsaparilla
was seldom given alone, but was used as a vehicle for the administration of mercury, iodide of potassium, and other powerful
and efficient drugs, so that it often obtained credit which it by

no means deserved. We believe that sarsaparilla itself is utterly
without effect upon the economy, and that its reputation as a
'blood purifier,' whatever that may mean, is all rubbish. There
is one thing to be said in its favour—if it does no good, it can do
no harm. If there is any one who still retains a latent belief in its
virtues, he may indulge himself with perfect safety, with the full
assurance that he will not suffer in any way, unless it be in
pocket. The decoction of sarsaparilla is made by steeping two
and a half ounces of sarsaparilla cut into small pieces in a pint and
a half of boiling water, and gradually evaporating it down to a
pint. The dose is anything under a bucketful.—*The Family
Physician*, 1883.

Sometimes the most ludicrous ideas are produced by the use of
the hemp. One of Bayard Taylor's friends imagined, whilst
under the influence of the drug, that he was a steam engine.
He suddenly sprang from his seat to the floor exclaiming, with
a shriek of the wildest laughter, 'Oh, ye gods! I'm a locomotive!'
This was his ruling hallucination, and for the space of two or
three hours he continued to pace to and fro, with a measured
stride, exhaling his breath in violent jets, and when he spoke
dividing his words into syllables, each of which he brought out
with a jerk, at the same time turning his hands at his sides as if
they were the cranks of imaginary wheels. The delusion must,
in this case, have been very perfect, for having raised a pitcher of
water to his lips, to quench his thirst, he put it down again
without drinking, exclaiming, in the greatest excitement, 'How
can I fill my boiler when I'm letting off steam?'—*The Cyclopaedia
of Practical Medicine*, 1833.

After a time the use of tar in the treatment of diseases was, in
this country, almost abandoned. There is no doubt that the
statements made as to its efficacy were greatly exaggerated, but
at the same time it must be admitted that tar is a very valuable
remedy for many complaints. It is of very great value in the
treatment of *winter cough, chronic bronchitis*, and *asthma*. It is
largely used for these complaints both in France and Belgium,
and patients who have tried it usually speak of it most enthusi-
astically. They say that by its use they are enabled to curtail the
duration and lessen the severity of their attacks, and there can

be no doubt that such is the case. An improvement is, as we can certify, usually noticeable in from four to seven days, it rapidly increases, and in about three weeks the cough is practically well.

There are several ways in which tar can be administered. We have already spoken of Berkeley's tar water. The French call it *eau de goudron*, and take it with sugar and water, or with claret at dinner, the combination being almost tasteless—a point of no small consideration with them. Anybody who would make a few gallons of tar water at the commencement of the winter for the benefit of the old people with coughs and colds would, we are sure, be doing them a service. They will not make any difficulty about taking it.—*Ibid.*

TO MAKE TAR-WATER

Pour a Gallon of cold Water on a Quart of Tar, stir and mix them thoroughly with a Ladle, or flat Stick, for three or four Minutes; after which let it stand 48 Hours, for the Tar to sink to the Bottom; then pour off the clear Water, and keep it in Bottles, well corked, for Use. To be taken about half a Pint Morning and Night, not eating for two Hours both before and after, and holding the Nostrils, whilst a Person drinks it, 'twill not be offensive.

No more Drink being to be made from the same Tar, it is as good as any for all common Uses, such as greasing of Coach or Cart Wheels, etc.—*The Lady's Companion*, 1751.

A Cure for the Gout, published by Thomas Sandford, and Edward Gent, both of the City of Kilkenny. Half an Ounce of Hiera-picra, and eight Grains of Cochineal, finely powder'd, being put into a Pint of the best Red-Port, let it stand at least 24 Hours, shake the Bottle well, and often, during that Time, but shake not the Bottle for three or four Hours before you draw off any of the Tincture for Use; take of this half a Quartern to near a Quartero, according as you find yourself strong or weak; you must continue taking of this every second, third, or fourth Day, 'till you take the whole Pint; and if the Gout returns, take another Pint as before, and so do to every Fit.

This Tincture, if taken in a Fit of the Gout, in a few Hours dissolves all the Particles in the Blood which causes the Pain, and if pursued, as before directed, will in Time work them all out of the Blood. It likewise carries off all new Swellings soon, and all old Swellings in Time; you may use Posset-Drink with this as with other Physick, yet if you take nothing after it, it will work very well; the properest Time of taking it is in the Morning fasting, or at Night, if you do not eat or drink for four or five Hours before; continue in Bed from the Time of taking it, 'till it purges you downwards, which will be in about twelve Hours Time; but if you have not a Stool in that Time, take a large Spoonful more.

If you have the Rheumatism or Sciatica, take the Tincture as before, but in a larger Quantity. I caution all People that take this, to have a special Care that they do not take Cold, for it will cause many to sweat greatly for a Time; and if they take Cold, they will be apt to be griped; which if they are, a little mulled Port-Wine, or a Spoonful of the Tincture, immediately eases them.—*Ibid.*

OF THE GOUT

In cases of gout nothing is more fatal than to hinder the Gouty Matter, now grown mature, and remaining unexpelled, as well as uncorrected by proper Medicines, from falling on the usual Parts, which indeed cause great Pain, but no Danger. If it invades the Brain, it will occasion Apoplexies, Palsies, a Delirium, Weaknesses, Dozing, Tremors, or universal Convulsions: If it attacks the Lungs, it produces an Asthma, a Cough or a Suffocation. If the Intercostals and Pleura, a convulsive Pleurisy: If the abdominal Viscera, Nauseas, Anxieties, Vomiting, Belching, Gripings, or Spasms of the Viscera. It is almost incredible how many diseases it creates, which are suddenly mortal; or at least not to be cured but by reviving the Fit of the Gout, which had been disturbed, and rendering it as severe as possible.

These last mentioned Evils happen from injudicious Applications of Narcotics, Refrigerants, Astringents, or Incrassants; or from Medicines which cause a Revulsion from the diseased Part, or from debilitating, evacuating, or suffocating Remedies. Hence Bleeding, Purging upwards or downwards, Plasters, Pultices, of the Nature abovementioned, and all Opiates produce these

Effects; as also a spontaneous Weakness brought on by extreme old Age; or from the extreme Parts being so obstructed, corrupted, withered, or perished, that the morbisic Matter cannot pass through them any longer.

To abate the excessive Pain in the Part affected, if there be an absolute Necessity, Opiates may be given internally, and the Patient may drink plentifully of hot Whey, or any other Liquor of the like Nature. External Emollients and Anodynes may be used laid on pretty hot, or the Part affected may be beat with Nettles.—*The General Practice of Physic*, 1763.

Dr Mead's Receipt for the Cure of the Bite of a Mad Dog. Let the Patient be blooded at the Arm nine or ten Ounces. Take of the Herb call'd in Latin, Lichen Cinereus Terrestris, in English, Ash-colour'd Ground Liverwort, clean'd dry'd, and powder'd, half an Ounce; and Black-Pepper powder'd, two Drams; mix these well together, and divide the Powder into four Doses, one of which must be taken every Morning, fasting, for four Mornings successively, in half a Pint of Cow's Milk warm. After these four Doses are taken, the Patient must go into the Cold Bath, or a cold Spring, or River, every Morning fasting, for a Month. He must be dipt all over, but not stay in (with his Head above Water) longer than half a Minute, if the Water be very cold. After this he must go in three Times a Week, for a Fortnight longer.

NB The Lichen is a very common Herb, and grows generally in sandy and barren Soils all over England. The right Time to gather it is in the Months of October and November.

Another Cure for the Bite of a Mad Dog, brought from Tonquin by Sir George Cobb, of Somersetshire, Bart. Take 24 Grains of Native Cinnabar, 24 Grains of Factitious Cinnabar, and 16 Grains of Musk; grind all these together into an exceeding fine Powder, and put it into a small Tea Cup of Arrack, Rum or Brandy; let it be well mix'd, and give it the Person as soon as possible, after the Bite; a Second Dose of the same must be repeated thirty Days after; and a Third may be taken in thirty Days more: But if the Symptoms of Madness appear on the Persons, they must take one of the above Doses immediately, and a second in an Hour after; and, if wanted, a third must be given a few Hours afterwards.

NB The above Recipe is calculated for a full grown Person, but must be given to Children in smaller Quantities, in Proportion to their Ages.

This Medicine has been given to Hundreds with Success, and Sir George Cobb himself has cured two Persons who had the Symptoms of Madness upon them.—*The Lady's Companion*, 1751.

12

Some Philosophic and Moral Problems Concerning the Practice of Physic

Every wise physician is a dogmatist, but a dogmatical physician is one of the most absurd animals that lives. We say he is a dogmatist in physic who employs his reason, and, from some acquaintance with the nature of the human body, thinks he can throw some light upon diseases, and ascertain the proper methods of cure; and I have known none who were not dogmatists except those who seemed to be incapable of reasoning or were too lazy for it.—*Eminent Doctors*, 1885.

The people have too long been educated to look upon a medical monopoly as the safest means of ensuring their health: they swallow nauseous drugs, but turn with indifference from vegetables as a medicine, while they eat them with complacency at their dinner: that which is thought excellent to sustain them in health, loses its power when they are prostrated by disease—such is the reasoning of prejudice, of the shallow and unthinking mind!—*Botanic Guide to Health*, 1859.

If we look back to the Origin of the Art of Medicine, we shall find its first Foundations to be owing to mere Chance, unforeseen Events, and natural Instinct. Nor does it appear there were in the Beginning any public Professors of this most useful Branch of Learning; for sick Persons were placed in Cross-ways, and other public Places, to receive the Advice of Passengers, who had Skill sufficient to direct them to an efficacious Remedy, suitable to their Disorder. And the better to preserve the Memory of any remarkable Cure, the Disease, the Remedy, and the Success, were engraved on Pillars, or written on the Walls of Temples, that Patients in the like Cases might have Recourse thereto for Instruction and Relief.

Hence it appears, that the Rise of this Art was owing to repeated Trials and long Experience, which gave an Insight into the Virtues of Herbs and Plants, Metals and Minerals; and in what Diseases they were attended with most Success.

Let none think that Medicines are to be given at random in every Stage of acute Diseases; for here the Physician's Judgment is absolutely necessary. And the seasonable Exhibition of a Remedy, after the Guidance of Nature, will always distinguish the able Practitioner from the dangerous Quack. For this Reason, I have been careful in reciting all the Symptoms of Diseases, and their natural Progress to Recovery or Death.

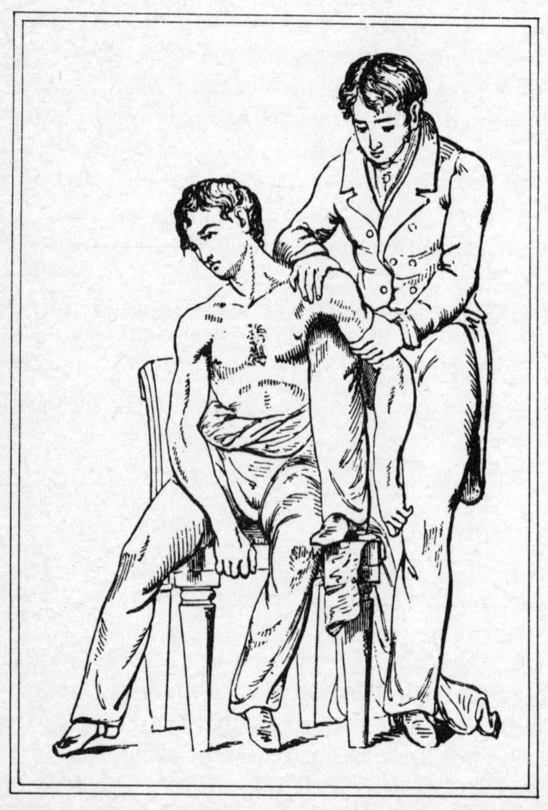

There is nothing I would recommend more to a Practitioner, than Affability and Sweetness of Temper, with Regard to the Patient, and to take all prudent Methods to keep up his Spirits;

nay, even when in a Disease it is necessary to wait to observe the Tendency of Nature, it will not be amiss to give innocent Trifles, to convince him he is not neglected. For when a sick Person is persuaded that he has a diligent and able Physician, that very Persuasion will contribute greatly to promote the Cure. On the other hand, there is nothing more dangerous than a fatal Prognostic; for this, instead of demonstrating superior Knowledge, too often either dejects the Patient and hastens his Exit, or proves the would-be Aesculapius to be a mere Medicaster, who perhaps would be better pleased with a sinister Event, than to see his Skill in Predictions baffled.—*The General Practice of Physic,* 1763.

It should be borne in mind that by disease we mean the sum total of certain morbid changes that take place within the body. The mistake is often made of supposing that disease is a something which has a distinct entity, that it is something that is taken into the body, and may be cast out again by appropriate remedies. You often hear patients, and even doctors, talk of 'driving the disease off through the kidneys,' or 'sweating it out of him.' Many people seem to regard disease as being something which has distinct physical properties, something that can be felt and seen. It is common enough to hear people say that 'he threw the disease off his stomach, just for all the world like a lump of currant jelly,' or for them to use some expression showing equally conclusively that they regard disease as having a distinct entity.— *The Family Physician,* 1883.

The common method of compounding and decompounding medicines, can never be reconciled to common sense. Experience shows, that one thing will cure most disorders, at least as well as twenty put together. Then why do you add the other nineteen? Only to swell the apothecary's bill! nay, possibly on purpose to prolong the distemper, that the doctor and he may divide the spoil.—*Hydropathy or the Cold Water Cure,* 1842.

No one seems to reflect that at least a doctor ought to be able to cure himself. We are so accustomed to illness and wretchedness, that we consider it a necessary part of this life, and are the less disposed to complain, since the masters of physic suffer very seriously from its effects themselves.—*Ibid.*

RELATING TO THE PATIENT

As a Man generally takes more Aliment than is necessary to generate Blood and Serum, and the common Excretions are not sufficient to carry off superfluous Humours, extraordinary ones sometimes happen at stated times; hence the bleeding Piles and Haemorrhages of the Nose, as also large Sweats, Loosenesses, Running at the Nose, Coughs, plentiful Spitting, all which tend to promote Health; and if these are defective or suppressed, dangerous Diseases may arise. Wherefore it is highly hazardous to suppress Secretions of this Kind. Hence great Passions of the Mind, especially Terror, which constringes the small Vessels, very cold Air, and sudden Refrigerating of the Body, produce dangerous Stagnations of the Fluids, and sudden and capital Disorders in the vital Motions. The same may be said of critical Excretions, if unadvisedly stopt; for they not only renew the Disease, but render it much more dangerous.

If the Mind is not composed and at Ease, but subject to various Passions and Commotions, Diseases are cured with greater Difficulty; therefore Enquiry is to be made whether the Patient is not addicted to hard Study, and to profound and fatiguing Meditations, which is common in those who apply themselves to the Sciences of Metaphysics and Mathematics, and are fond of nocturnal Lucubrations; for intense Thinking consumes the Spirits, and brings on a Weakness of the Brain and nervous Parts; whence they are subject to dangerous Diseases of the Head, namely, Apoplexy, Melancholy, Madness, and Weakness of Memory.

It can hardly be imagined what a Consent there is between the Brain and its Membranes, between the Stomach and the adjoining Intestines, they being greatly nervous, and induced with an exquisite Sense; whence many Students are troubled with a bad Digestion, Costiveness, and the hypochondriac Passion.—*The General Practice of Physic*, 1763.

The advantages which attend 'change of air,' in the treatment of

MR. HOOPER'S IMPROVED
HYDROSTATIC BEDS,
OR MATTRESSES AND CUSHIONS,
FOR PLACING ON AN ORDINARY BEDSTEAD.
ANY TEMPERATURE MAY BE USED.

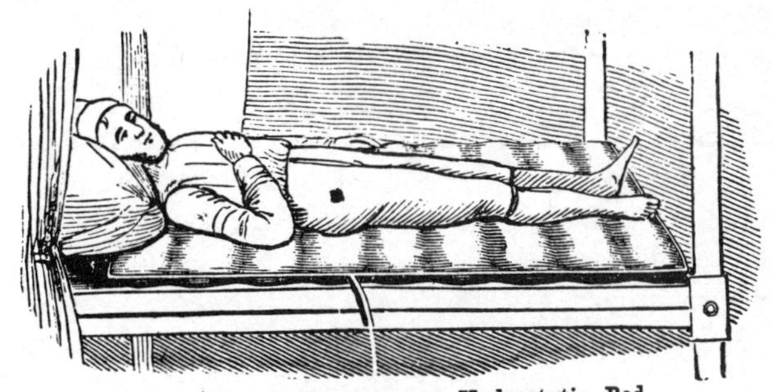

The Full-length Mattress or Hydrostatic Bed.
The width of the Bed should be sent with the Order.

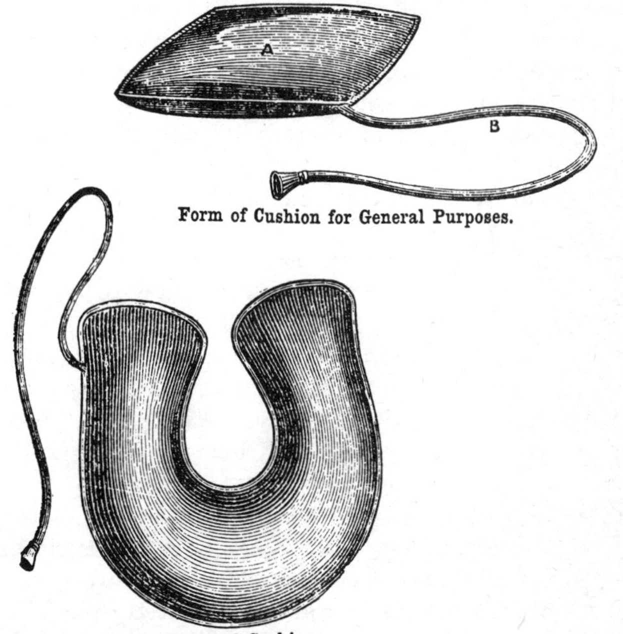

Form of Cushion for General Purposes.

Horse-Shoe Shaped Cushion.

various diseases, have been ascribed by many physicians to the exhilarating impressions thus produced upon the mind, and to the simultaneous change of habits which usually takes place upon such occasions.

It therefore follows that, in the recommendation of a place of resort for invalids, various circumstances are to be taken into consideration: it is no less important to furnish amusement for the mind, than to provide salubrious air and wholesome food for the body. A continual change of residence is, perhaps, better adapted for insuring our object, than a protracted stay in any one place.

This truth is beautifully illustrated by an anecdote related by Sydenham, and will go further in establishing the importance of the principle I am desirous of enforcing, than any argument which it is in my power to adduce. This great physician, having long attended a gentleman of fortune with little or no advantage, frankly avowed his inability to render him any further service, adding, at the same time, that there was a physician of the name of Robinson, at Inverness, who had distinguished himself by the performance of many remarkable cures of the same complaint as that under which his patient laboured, and expressing a conviction that, if he applied to him, he would come back cured. This was too encouraging a proposal to be rejected: the gentleman received from Sydenham a statement of his case; with the necessary letter of introduction, and proceeded without delay to the place in question.

On arriving at Inverness, and anxiously inquiring for the residence of Dr Robinson, he found, to his utter dismay and disappointment, that there was no physician of that name in the place, nor ever had been in the memory of any person there. The gentleman returned, vowing eternal hostility against the peace of Sydenham; and on his arrival at home, instantly expressed his indignation, in not very measured terms, at having been sent so many hundred miles for no purpose. 'Well,' replies Sydenham, 'are you better in health?'—'Yes; I am now perfectly well, but no thanks to you.'—'No?' says Sydenham, 'but you may thank Dr Robinson for curing you. I wished to send you a journey with some object of interest in view: I knew it would be of service to you: in going, you had Dr Robinson and his wonderful cures in contemplation, and in returning you were equally engaged in thinking of scolding me.'—*A Treatise on Diet*, 1837.

Alas! our modern mercenary Tribe,
But scarce observe their Patient—and prescribe—
For who can spend his Time and tamely wait,
To hear the Sick Man's Tale, or Nurse's Chat
No *Doctor* then would have it in his Power
To see above—two Patients—in an Hour!
No more wou'd swell th' Apothecary's Bill,
With nauseous Bole, pearl Julep, gilded Pill,
Cardiac Drops or Mixtures swallow'd down,
And *ter in Die* Draughts—each—half a Crown.

A Physical Rhapsody, 1751.

Appendix One

*In which are exposed Some Feigned Diseases,
followed by Some Most Instructive Proverbs and
Aphorisms concerning the Attainment and Retention
of Good Health*

Diseases are most frequently feigned among soldiers and sailors to avoid duty and to obtain exemption from service; and by the beggar to gain sympathy, and thus obtain the fruitful harvest of alms he often reaps. Others often do the same to obtain better diet; prisoners to be exempt from prison labours; whilst yet another and not uncommon class of feigned diseases are those in young women of an hysterical turn, who desire to obtain the sympathy of friends and neighbours.

A good classification of feigned diseases is into fictitious and factitious; the former having no real existence; the latter having real existence, but being of artificial and voluntary origin; for it is wonderful what tortures malingerers will inflict upon themselves or voluntarily undergo in order that they may attain their end. Frequently, among bodies of men, such attempts at imposture become epidemic, and can only be got rid of by sharp measures. No fixed order will be here observed, but the above distinctions may be borne in mind.

Swellings of various kinds are often produced by soldiers and prisoners; they tie a piece of string tightly round the arm or leg, and so a swelling resembling dropsy is produced. Such are easily discovered by watching the supposed patient for an hour or two, when its effects will have disappeared, and no swelling be left. Windy swelling of the abdomen (tympanitis) is easily simulated by swallowing air, and as easily got rid of by a stiff dose of turpentine and castor oil. As for sores, manufactured or feigned, their name is legion. Ulcers of all kinds are favourite subjects of simulation. Corrosive substances are applied to a part either before or after the skin has been otherwise removed, and the sore thus formed is prevented from healing by similar means.

Skin diseases are also frequently feigned. Ophthalmia is very frequently manufactured among soldiers. All kinds of irritants are used, and the right eye is generally the one affected. Vomiting is frequently simulated, especially by women. The habit, once induced, is easily kept up, and, of course, should lead to emaciation and an appearance of disease. Most frequently, though not always, this is not the case when feigned. Diarrhœa is also most frequently simulated by women, who will introduce all kinds of things into their motions. Alterations of the urine have been tried to be passed off in a similar manner; and gonorrhœa has been feigned sometimes with the worst intent. Blood spitting—hæmoptysis—is a favourite disease among simulating females. Sucking the gums will generally induce it, and it is not easy to detect it. Careful watching will usually elicit the truth.

Epilepsy or convulsions of any kind are favourite subjects of study and practice among rogues of the mendicant class. Among those who have much to do with such rascals there is a rather effectual, as being very powerful, way of detecting them. This is by thrusting some sharp body under the finger nail of the malingerer. It is not pleasant, but is generally effectual. Paralysis of all kinds is frequently feigned, but it needs a skilful impostor to escape detection. Very frequently this is easy; the physician makes an aside remark not intended for the patient's ear, stating that such and such a symptom is not quite as usual. Having taken care to state the reverse of what is actually the fact, he will generally find not long after that the symptom has appeared exactly as he pretended to say it ought.

Deafness and dumbness have often been feigned, sometimes with singular success. Blindness of various kinds and degrees are frequently feigned. Short-sight used to be frequently feigned in the army among recruits. This was detected by giving him long-sight glasses to read with. Of course, had he been short-sighted, this with such glasses would have been impossible. Usually the trick succeeded. Jaundice has sometimes been tried, as, indeed, have most diseases. Staining the skin with saffron or rhubarb was the commonest form of deception. Affections of the mind are very frequently assumed by criminals.—*Household Medicine,* 1892.

PROBLEMS AND APHORISMS OF HEALTH

Old young and old long.

More die by food than famine.

Be temperate in all things.

Eat a bit before you drink.

Be not solitary; be not idle.

Eat at pleasure, drink by measure.

Who goes to bed supperless, all night tumbles and tosses.

Diet cures more than the lancet.

After dinner sit a while, after supper walk a mile.

He that goes to bed thirsty rises healthy.

You should not touch your eye but with your elbow.

The best physicians are Dr Diet, Dr Quiet and Mr Merryman.

'Tis good to walk till the blood appears in the cheek, but not the sweat on the brow.

The excesses of our youth are drafts upon our old age, payable with interest, about thirty years after date.

The rule for the rich man to be healthy is by exercise and abstinence to live as if he were poor.

'Nor love thy life nor hate; but what thou livest
  Live well; how long or short, permit to heaven.'

We seldom repent of having eaten too little.

Better lose a supper than gain a hundred physicians.

One hour's sleep before midnight is worth two after.

The head and feet keep warm; the rest will take no harm.

A good surgeon must have an eagle's eye, a lion's heart, and a lady's hand.

God never made his work for man to mend.

In general, mankind, since the improvement of cookery, eat twice as much as nature requires.

The patient can oftener do without the doctor than the doctor without the patient.

Causing a symptom to disappear is very seldom the cure of any human infirmity. The true course is to prevent the symptom.

Many a pie has cost an industrious husband a twenty-pound note in doctors' bills; and many a human life has paid for an apple dumpling.

All sick people want to get well, but not always in the best way. Said a wealthy man, 'Doctor, strike at the root of the disease,' and smash went the decanter under the faithful physician's hand.

The loss of our strength is much oftener occasioned by the vices of our youth than the ravages of age; it is early intemperance and licentiousness that consign to old age a worn out constitution.

In these days, half of our diseases come from the neglect of the body in the overwork of the brain. In this railway age, the wear and tear of labour and intellect go on without pause or self pity. We live longer than our forefathers, but we suffer more from a thousand artificial anxieties and cares. They fatigued only the muscles but we exhaust the finer strength of the nerves.

Appendix Two

*In Which is Described a Selection of Gymnastic
Exercises Conducive to Physical and Mental
Health and Vigour*

Physical education has, to a very great extent, been left, in this country, to take care of itself. We are no worshippers of the system which would subordinate mind to matter, which would make a well-trained boating-man or cricketer the most perfect being on earth, but assuredly we do not hold to the other view, that men may grow up misshapen, rickety articles, provided only their mental powers are developed to the uttermost. Strength of body is necessary to strength of mind, and most men of great mental vigour, not necessarily of subtlety and refinement, are also men of bodily vigour. Here it may be as well to say that physical education does not mean what is sometimes described as 'hardening' children. You see a miserable little wretch, shivering in the cold of winter, only half dressed, and you are told by his parents they are hardening him. Well, it is true the result may be satisfactory, but it may not; some live and do well, but a good many die in the process. Physical education means taking the material you have got, however unpromising, and making the best of it. To do so, you require good food and clothing, air and exercise, and the cleanliness which comes after godliness.

For giving strength to the chest, fencing is a good exercise, and the same is to be said of the Indian club exercise. Shuttlecock, as an exercise which calls into play the muscles of the trunk, chest and arms, is also very beneficial. After a little practice, it can be played with the left as easily as with the right hand, and is, therefore, very useful in preventing curvature and giving vigour to the spine in young women. It is an excellent plan to play with a battledore in each hand, and to strike with them alternately. Lawn-tennis and badminton, to speak of more elaborate games, deserve also the highest praise on the score of health, and it is to be

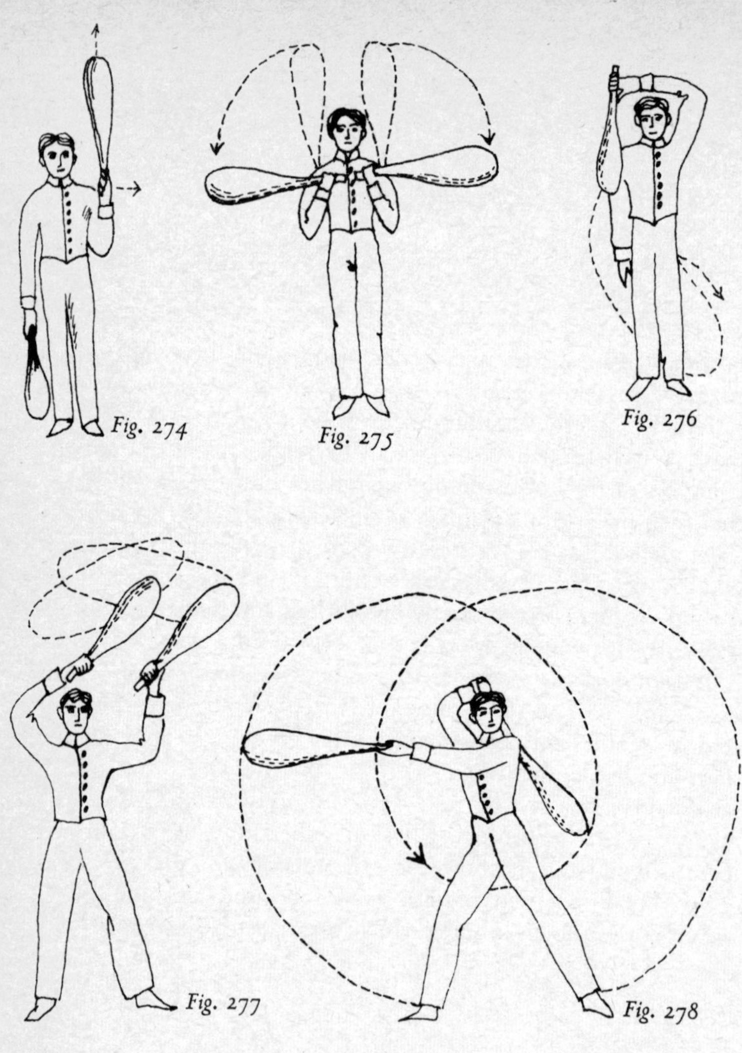

Fig. 274   Fig. 275   Fig. 276

Fig. 277   Fig. 278

hoped that they will enjoy a long-lived popularity. The now declining croquet might also well be granted a new lease of life.

From figs. 274–78, drawn from Captain Crawley's *Handbook on Gymnastics*, the reader will obtain a good idea of the nature of Indian club exercises.

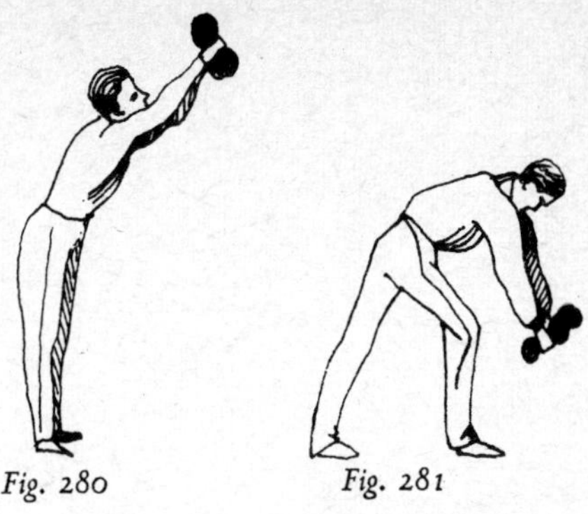

Fig. 280   Fig. 281

First, then, we take up the bells. The raising and swinging of the bells take place from the standing position. Stoop, seize both bells, recover the upright position, and raise them above the head. Repeat this by lowering the bells to the ground, bending the knees, and then rising to the upright position, as shown in figs. 280 and 281.

Moving the bells in horizontal and slanting planes forms the next exercise. These are better explained in the diagrams (figs. 282–285) than by any amount of verbal description.

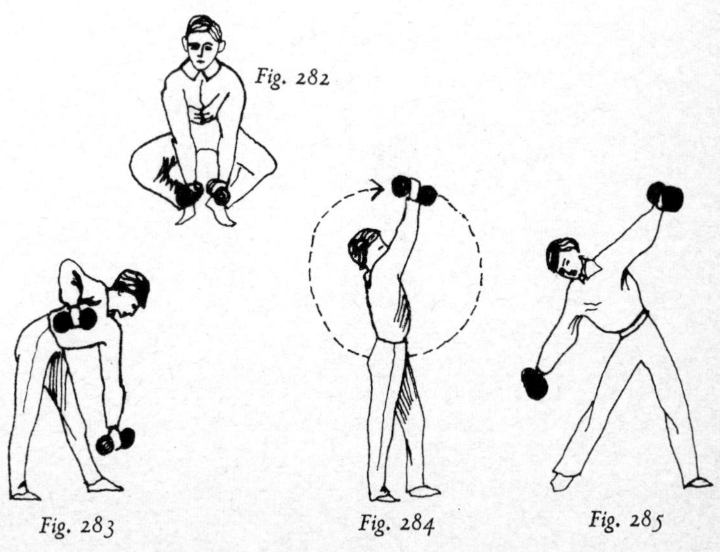

Fig. 282

Fig. 283   Fig. 284   Fig. 285

CALISTHENICS

As a preliminary course to regular gymnastics pupils are generally practised in the simple movements known as Calisthenics, or movements without implements. These exercises are equally fitted for both sexes, and their importance as promoters of health can hardly be over-estimated.

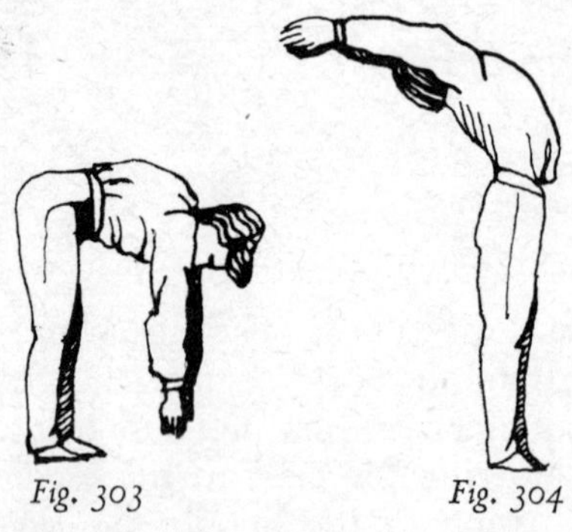

Fig. 303   Fig. 304

Stretch the arms upwards, with the palms of the hands facing each other, and keep the legs perfectly stiff. Then bend forward, and, with the knees still quite firm, touch the ground with the tips of the fingers (fig. 303). From this position swing backwards to the back bend (fig. 304).

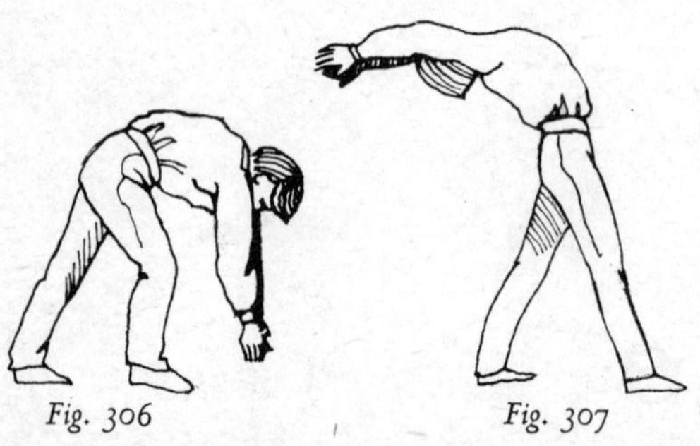

Fig. 306   Fig. 307

Advance the right leg about eighteen inches and stretch the arms upwards. Bend from this position to touch the ground with the tips of the fingers (fig. 306); then bend backwards (fig. 307). Exactly the same movements should be repeated with the left leg advanced.

SOURCES

Extracts and Anecdotes have been obtained from the following sources:

The Family Physician, by Physicians and Surgeons of the Principal London Hospitals, 1883.
Pilgrimages to the Spas, James Johnson, M.D., 1841.
Sexual Physiology, R. T. Trall, 1866.
A Treatise on Diet, J. A. Paris, M.D., F.R.S., 1837.
My Water Cure, Sebastian Kneipp, 1892.
Diseases of the Rectum and Anus, E. D. Silver, M.D., 1851.
Hydropathy or The Cold Water Cure, as practised by Vincent Priessnitz, by R. T. Claridge Esq., 1842.
Eminent Doctors—Their Lives and Work, G. T. Bettany, 1885.
The Cyclopaedia of Practical Medicine, edited by John Forbes, Alexander Tweedie, John Conolly, 1833.
Hints to Husbands, George Morant, 1857.
Public Characters of 1800–1801, Lettsoms.
The Anatomy of Melancholy, Robert Burton, 1621.
On Consumption, Coughs, Colds, Asthma, R. J. Culverwell, M.D., 1834.
A Guide to Domestic Hydrotherapeia, James Manby Gully, M.D., 1863.
New Curative Treatment of Disease, M. Platen, 1901.
Practical Cases and Observations in Surgery, Dale Ingram, 1751.
An Essay towards a Complete New System of Midwifery, John Bunton, 1751.
The Lady's Companion, 1751.
Till the Doctor Comes, George H. Hope, M.D., M.R.C.S.E., 1870.
Botanic Guide to Health, A. I. Coffin, 1859.
An Essay Concerning the Effects of Air on Human Bodies, John Arbuthnot, 1733.
Eminent Doctors, their Lives and their Work, G. T. Bettany, 1751.
A Physical Rhapsody, Anon., 1751.
Notes on Nursing, Mrs. W. E. Gladstone.
The General Practice of Physic, R. Brookes, M.D., 1763.

West Wickham Cookery Book, 1934.
Gardener's Household Medicine and Sick Room Guide, 1898.
Household Medicine, George Black, M.B., Edin., 1892.
Dr. Paris on Diet and Regimen, 1837.
Theatrum Botanicum, John Parkinson, 1640.
Dangers to Health, T. Pridgin Teale, 1883.

Illustrations have been obtained from the above books and the following sources:

The Lancet, issues dated October 24, November 7, December 12, December 26 1857, January 18, February 22, March 8 and August 30 1873, May 23 1874.